Intermittent Fasting:

Lose Weight and Gain Muscle While Extending Your Lifespan and Leading A More Productive, Healthier Life!

Kevin Moore © 2017

All rights reserved. No part of this book may be reproduced in any form without permission in writing from the author. Reviewers may quote brief passages in reviews.

Disclaimer:

This book is for informational purposes only and the author, his agents, heirs, and assignees do not accept any responsibilities for any liabilities, actual or alleged, resulting from the use of this information.

This report is not "professional advice." The author encourages the reader to seek advice from a professional where any reasonably prudent person would do so. While every reasonable attempt has been made to verify the information contained in this eBook, the author and his affiliates cannot assume any responsibility for errors, inaccuracies or omissions, including omissions in transmission or reproduction.

Any references to people, events, organizations, or business entities are for educational and illustrative purposes only, and no intent to falsely characterize, recommend, disparage, or injure is intended or should be so construed. Any results stated or implied are consistent with general results, but this means results can and will vary. The author, his agents, and assigns, make no promises or guarantees, stated or implied. Individual results will vary and this work is supplied strictly on an "at your own risk" basis.

Introduction

Thanks for grabbing my book "Intermittent Fasting: Lose Weight and Gain Muscle While Extending Your Lifespan and Leading A More Productive, Healthier Life!" By reading this guide you've decided that you're interested in uncovering all the benefits that Intermittent Fasting can have on improving your health and overall well-being. I'm not going to lie and say this is the easiest path to go down. It's not! It will take both hard work and dedication on your part to achieve your goals, especially in the beginning stages. However, after a slight readjustment period, you'll begin to feel lighter and healthier than you have in years.

This book will teach you everything you need to know to begin Intermittent Fasting. I'll be going over the major concepts behind the process and popular methods you can use to fast safely and effectively. I've also included a full resource guide with links to tools, apps, resources, and books to help you along your journey. If that's not enough I've also packed this guide with over 70+ healthy low-calorie meals to get you started in the right direction.

I'm excited to get started. Let's dive in!

Chapter One: Intermittent Fasting Basics

What is Intermittent Fasting?

Intermittent Fasting (IF) is one of the biggest fitness and health trends sweeping the nation. People love it so much because it allows one to improve their health and lose weight following a simple lifestyle. There are a ton of studies that show it has an incredible effect on your brain and body. Many studies also believe it will help to extend your lifespan. Intermittent Fasting refers to an eating pattern that cycles between both periods of eating and fasting. Intermittent Fasting doesn't tell you what foods you need to eat but when you should be eating them. It's not a conventional diet like the Atkins Diet or Ketogenic Diet. It would be more aptly described as a change in your eating patterns.

A few of the most popular Intermittent Fasting methods involve either fasting for 16 hours a day with an 8 eight period where you're allowed to eat or fasting for 24 hours at a time 2 different days a week. Fasting dates back thousands of years. It was often done by our ancestors because food wasn't as readily available. It makes a lot of sense when you think about it as our ancestors didn't have access to such conveniences as supermarkets or refrigerated food. When food wasn't available our bodies began to evolve so they could function for extended periods of time without food. For many people, fasting is considered more natural than eating multiple meals spread out at the same time every day.

Fasting has also played a major role in many religions throughout the centuries, including Buddhism, Christianity, and Islam. Many followers of these faiths would integrate fasting into part of their daily lives as a sign of devotion to their deities. To this day fasting still plays a part in these faiths, showing the longevity and power behind it.

When you choose to fast, a lot of things begin to occur in your body on both a molecular and cellular level. For example, your body will change its hormone levels in order to make stored up body fat accessible. The cells in your body will also begin to start up critical repair processes and will even change up the expression of your genes.

<u>Here are a just a few of the changes that will occur in your body when you begin to fast:</u>

Gene Expression - Changes occur in the function of your genes related to protection from disease and longevity.

Insulin - The insulin sensitivity in your body improves and the actual levels of insulin begin to drop in dramatic fashion. Having lower insulin levels makes the fat stored in your body more accessible.

Cellular Repair - When fasting, your cells will begin to initiate the cellular repair process. This includes autophagy, which is when your cells digest and remove any old and defective proteins that have built up inside your cells.

Human Growth Hormone (HGH) - Your levels of growth hormone will increase as much as 5 times what they are currently. This benefits you both in the muscle gain department and fat loss department.

The changes I describe above are the primary things responsible for all the different health benefits associated with Intermittent Fasting.

The primary reason most people try Intermittent Fasting is to lose weight. The idea is that by eating fewer meals you'll be automatically reducing the number of calories you're taking in. Also, fasting helps to change your hormone levels to speed up the weight loss process. Intermittent Fasting not only leads to these increased growth hormone levels and lower insulin, it also increases the amount of norepinephrine you release. For those of you that don't know norepinephrine is a fat burning hormone. Studies have shown that because of all these hormonal changes triggered by fasting you can increase your bodies metabolic rate by between 3% and 14%.

Eating less and consuming fewer calories along with burning more calories due to hormonal changes mean Intermittent Fasting affects both sides of a person's calories equation leading to weight loss. When compared to most other types of weight studies, Intermittent Fasting stacks up quite well. Studies show that Intermittent Fasting helps reduce the amount of dangerous belly fat that can build up around a person's organs and lead to a variety of different diseases. Remember, that if you binge while fasting your results won't be very good. Eating fewer calories is one of the hallmarks of Intermittent Fasting. Learn to eat sensibly during the hours you're allowed to eat and you'll watch the weight begin to drop off in no time.

Popular Intermittent Fasting Methods

The 16/8 Method - Also known as the Leangains protocol, this method involves you skipping breakfast and then restricting your daily eating schedule to a period of only 8 hours. For example, eating only from 12 pm to 8 pm. Then you fast for the remaining 16 hours in between.

Eat-Stop-Eat - This method involves fasting for a period of 24 hours, once or twice every week. For example, not eating from dinnertime on one day until dinnertime on the next day.

The 5:2 Diet - This method involves fasting on two non-consecutive days each week, only eating a total of 500 to 600 calories. For the rest of the week, you would eat a normal sensible diet.

By forcing yourself to consume fewer calories, all of these fasting methods will help you lose weight as long as you're not compensating by eating too much during the allowed eating periods. Personally, I tried them all and ended up following the 16/8 method long term. I found it to be the easiest and most sustainable method to stick to. That's probably why it's also the most popular method. Bottom line, there are many Intermittent Fasting methods. All of them split your day or your week into separate "fasting periods" and "eating periods."

Health Benefits of Intermittent Fasting

Anti-Aging - Intermittent Fasting has been shown to extend the lifespan in rats. Studies concluded that fasted rats would live between 36% to 83% longer.

Brain Health - Intermittent Fasting has been shown to increase the brain hormone known as BDNF, which may aid in the growth of new nerve cells. Fasting has also been shown to protect against Alzheimer's disease.

Cancer - Studies in animals suggest that Intermittent Fasting can help to prevent cancer from occurring.

Heart Health - Intermittent fasting has been shown to reduce blood triglycerides, LDL cholesterol, insulin resistance, blood sugar, and inflammatory markers. These are all considered serious risk factors for heart disease.

Inflammation - Studies have shown reductions in inflammation markers is a key driver of a lot of different chronic diseases.

Insulin resistance - Intermittent Fasting can help to reduce our insulin resistance, lowering your blood sugar by between 3% and 6% and our fasting insulin levels by between 20% and 30%. This can help to protect us against diseases such as type 2 diabetes.

Weight Loss - Intermittent Fasting can help aid in weight loss and belly fat reduction. It can do this without the need to consciously restrict your caloric intake.

Most of this research is still in preliminary stages. The majority of these studies were smaller in scope and limited to animals. The results, however, are hopeful and demand greater research. Intermittent Fasting is not something that is meant for everyone. People who have suffered from eating disorders or are underweight shouldn't be Intermittent Fasting without the consent of a doctor. The same goes for women who are trying to conceive, already pregnant, or currently breastfeeding. Intermittent Fasting can be dangerous when done under the wrong conditions.

Some studies suggest that Intermittent Fasting is more beneficial for men than it is for women. Studies have shown that Intermittent Fasting improves insulin sensitivity in males but made blood sugar control in women worse. It was also shown in studies involving rats to make the females infertile and cause them to miss their cycles. Just a few things to consider before starting this form of fasting. I always recommend consulting your physician first regardless of age, health, or gender. They'll be able to help you make a sound medical decision regarding your health.

Safety and Side Effects of Intermittent Fasting

The primary side effect related to Intermittent Fasting is hunger. When people begin fasting they often feel weaker and their mind feels like it isn't as sharp as they're used to. These feelings are temporary glitches as your body needs time to adapt and adjust to your new eating schedule.

If you're suffering from any of the medical conditions I've listed below you'll need to check with your doctor to make sure this type of fast is right for you. Don't let this list scare you off. Intermittent Fasting has an excellent safety profile. There's nothing inherently dangerous about following an intermittent eating schedule as long as you stay well nourished and are in general good health.

Blood Sugar Regulation Issues

Breastfeeding

Diabetes

Female Trying to Conceive

Female With Amenorrhea

History of Eating Disorders

Low Blood Pressure

Pregnant

Underweight

Taking Medications

Intermittent Fasting Frequently Asked Questions

Here are answers to the most common questions about intermittent fasting.

1. Can I drink liquids during the fast?

Yes. Drinking water, tea, coffee, and other beverages with no calories is acceptable. Don't add any sugar to your coffee. A tiny amount of cream or milk can be alright. Coffee tends to be beneficial when fasting as it helps to blunt your hunger.

2. Isn't it unhealthy to skip breakfast?

No. Skipping meals even breakfast have been shown to actually have the opposite effect as long as you're maintaining a healthy diet overall.

3. Can I take supplements while fasting?

Yes. Remember, that some types of supplements (fat-soluble vitamins) will work more effectively when had with your meals.

4. Will fasting slow down my metabolism?

No. Studies have shown that short-term fasts, such as those found in Intermittent Fasting, will actually help boost your metabolism. On the flip side, longer fasts (lasting 3 days or more) can help to suppress your metabolism.

5. Will fasting cause muscle loss?

It can. Every type of weight loss method can cause a person to lose muscle. That is why it's important to continue lifting weights and take in a high amount of protein. Studies have shown that Intermittent Fasting causes less muscle loss than if you were restricting your calories as you would in a regular diet.

6. Can I work out while fasting?

Yes. Working out while fasting is fine. Many people recommend taking a branched-chain amino acid (BCAAs) before engaging in a fasted workout.

7. Should kids fast?

No. That's a bad idea. Kids are still growing and have a different set of nutritional needs than adults. It's best not to mess with that.

How to Get Started

Chances are good that you've inadvertently already completed many "Intermittent Fasts" during your life. If you've ever had an early dinner, then slept in late and not eaten until lunchtime the next day, you've completed a 16 hour fast. Many people actually eat this way more often than they realize. This is especially true of people who don't feel hungry in the morning and wait until later in the day to have their first meal.

Personally, I've found that the 16/8 method is both the simplest and also the most sustainable way to do Intermittent Fasting long-term. I recommend trying this method out first and then switching to one of the other ones if it doesn't feel right for your lifestyle. If you find that the 16/8 method is easy and you feel good during your fast, you can try to move on to more advanced fasts like fasting 24 hours 1 to 2 times per week (Eat-Stop-Eat) or only eating approximately 500 to 600 calories 1 to 2 days each week (5:2 Diet). Another approach is to simply fast whenever you find it convenient. For example, skip a meal from time to time when you're not feeling hungry or don't have enough time to cook.

I recommend experimenting with the different types of approaches and find something that you not only enjoy but also fits into your schedule.

Chapter Two: Types of Intermittent Fasting & Fasting Schedules

6 Intermittent Fasting Methods

In this chapter, I'm going to go over 6 popular methods of Intermittent Fasting. There is no right way or wrong way among these methods. It's more of which way works best for you. All of these have been shown to be effective, it all depends on the individual to determine which one fits with your specific lifestyle the best.

1. The 16/8 Method

My top choice and also the most popular method being used. The 16/8 method involves you fasting each day for 14 to 16 hours and restricting your eating windows each day to between 8 to 10 hours. Within these eating windows, you can easily fit in 2 to 3 meals if not more. This method also can be referred to as the Leangains protocol. The majority of people favor this form of Intermittent Fasting because it's as simple as not eating anything after you've had dinner and skipping breakfast the next morning. For example, finishing your dinner at 7pm and then not eating anything until 11 am the next day. That 16-hour window between meals is considered a fast. For women, it's recommended that you fast for only 14 to 15 hours. Studies have shown that their system responds better to a slightly shorter fasting period.

For people used to eating a big breakfast each morning this method of fasting might take more getting used to at first. You can still drink coffee, water or other beverages with no calories during this time frame. I would definitely suggest doing so as it can help to curb your hunger significantly. Remember, once you're allowed to eat try sticking to healthy foods. If you gorge yourself on junk food and desserts you'll still take in an excessive amount of calories. The whole idea is to reduce the amount of time you're eating each day to also help naturally reduce the number of calories you're consuming.

After a small adjustment period, I've found this method of Intermittent Fasting to be almost effortless. I try to stick to a low-carb diet and I have a few beverages each morning to help curb any hunger pangs I might be feeling. I generally have my first meal between 12pm and 1pm and my last meal around 8pm and 9pm. Overall, I eat 3 meals each day. I have a smaller breakfast and lunch followed by a larger dinner. I might fit in a healthy snack once in a while or skip the lunch meal if I'm busy that day. I always make it a point not to skip my last meal as I don't want to throw my body off course. I know if I go to bed without that last meal I'll have to suffer through the next morning hungry in order to maintain the eating windows I've set for myself. I always try and eat at least a few hours before my bedtime in order to give my food some time to digest.

<u>Here's an example of my eating schedule.</u>

<u>*Eating Schedule:*</u>

Get up at 9am.

Breakfast at 12-1pm.

Lunch at 3-4pm.

Dinner at 8-9pm.

By skipping out on having a morning breakfast you force your body to begin breaking into its fat stores to help fuel itself instead of burning food for energy. This is why many people consider Intermittent Fasting the best fat loss diet available for both men and women. By pushing back your first meal later in the day you can enjoy bigger, more satisfying healthy meals while still staying at a caloric deficit.

Should You Be Drinking Coffee While Intermittent Fasting?

Consuming between 2 to 3 cups of coffee while your fasting has been shown to reduce appetite, accelerate metabolism, and give you a feeling of wellness. If you're planning on incorporating an exercise routine into your daily schedule then consuming coffee will have a positive impact on your overall stamina and strength.

My favorite kind of Intermittent Fasting coffee for burning fat and reducing my appetite is Fasting Fuel. I drink the stuff almost every day. The positive effects of coffee seem to last approximately 6 hours so even if you decide to train later in the day you'll still be able to get an extra boost from your morning coffee. Furthermore, coffee has been shown to be a great source of antioxidants and is known to have many other health benefits.

Breaking Your Fast

I suggest keeping your first two meals of the Intermittent Fasting meal plan extremely healthy and modestly sized. If you break your fast by consuming a large meal you'll shift your body out of its current sympathetic mode and into a parasympathetic mode. Doing so will shut off any fat burning and make you feel sluggish and tired. This type of feeling is definitely not an ideal way to spend your afternoon. Moreover, having a large meal during the middle of the day doesn't seem to be effective at curbing hunger (this is my own experience, things could be different for you). Lastly, having to cook and clean up after a big meal during the day can be a bit of a hassle and is often not very convenient.

Here is one example of an Intermittent Fasting meal plan. The goal behind this meal plan is to consume enough food to nourish your body and curb hunger without overtaxing your digestive system. Following a meal plan like this will let you maximize your energy and achieve sharper focus throughout the day. I prefer to have a small meal of between 300 to 400 calories. I opt for some fruit, protein, and healthy fats.

<u>*Example For 1st & 2nd Meals of Your Day:*</u>

Option #1: Chicken Breast, 1 Apple, Salad Greens, and Half an Avocado.

Option #2: 1 cup of Unsweetened Almond Milk mixed with 40 grams of Whey Protein, 20 grams of Almonds and 1 serving of Fruit.

Option #3: Cottage Cheese or Greek Yogurt topped with Almonds and Berries.

Option #4: 1 can of Tuna, 1 Apple, and 1 tablespoon of Olive Oil.

Option #5: Omelette (2 eggs + 1 cup of whites) and Berries.

As you can tell the sample meals included all have a source of fruit, protein, and healthy fats. This particular type of combination is something I've found to be extremely effective for remaining satisfied when consuming lower-calorie meals. The fruit is important because besides being very nutritious it's also easy to digest and is great for replenishing our liver glycogen. This is important because when you increase your liver glycogen you help bring yourself into an anabolic state which will help to reduce the feeling of hunger. Having a fat source with each meal also provides a similar result in the curbing of hunger. I've found when you skip out on having a healthy fat with each meal you become hungrier much quicker than when you have a meal that contains one.

Option #1: Steak, Sweet Potato, 1 serving of Vegetables.

Option #2: Chicken Breast, Potato Wedges (Boil 5 minutes and cook on a skillet in 2 to 3 teaspoons of oil), and 1 serving of Vegetables.

Option #3: Chicken Breast, Brown Rice, 1 serving of Vegetables, and Coconut Oil (add 1 to 3 teaspoons to your rice and 1 teaspoon for cooking chicken).

At this point in the day, you've already been fasting and have only consumed two smaller sized meals leaving yourself with a nice calorie buffer. I try to keep my first two meals of the day between 600 to 800 calories in total. Depending on your goal weight or reason for fasting these numbers may be slightly different for you. It's all about tailoring things to your specific set of needs. This particular way of doing things allows me to have a final meal for the day that is around 1000 calories. I found that this size meal will keep me going until the next day when I'm allowed to eat again.

For this meal, I like to go with something that contains a high amount of protein and a moderate amount of carbs and fat. If you're eating leaner protein like chicken you can still use things like butter with your rice and potatoes. However, if you're eating a fattier cut of meat such as salmon or beef I would suggest that you don't consume any more fats.

2. The 5:2 Diet

The 5:2 Diet is another popular form of Intermittent Fasting that involves a person eating like they normally would 5 days each week while reducing their calories to between 500 and 600 a day on the other 2 days of the week. This diet is also often referred to as the Fast Diet. It is recommended that women eat closer to the 500 calories mark, while men stick closer to the 600 calorie mark a day. For example, you might eat regularly on all days except Tuesdays and Fridays, where you would only consume two smaller sized meals each day.

Maximum flavor while consuming minimum calories

Fast days and eating carbs simply don't mix. Having a sugary donut will consume most of your caloric allowance and leave you feeling starved by later that evening. You should instead focus on salads, vegetables, and smaller servings of fish, lean meat, tofu, or eggs. This might feel a little plain and boring after the first few weeks so I recommend jazzing things up with some different spices, herbs, and flavorings. Try using curry pastes or chili flakes when cooking stews, soups, or beans. When eating salads try dressing things up with lemon juice or flavored vinegar. I found that eating a lot of soups on my fasting days helped keep me full longer. Try experimenting until you discover what works for you.

Experiment with your meal times

When trying to figure out when to eat on your fasting days I've found that the answer is usually different for everyone. I like to eat in the middle of the day and at the end of the day. However, I know many prefer eating in the morning and later at night because it makes them feel less hungry. Try out a few different meal times to see what you're comfortable with. There's been some evidence that suggests that the longer you can leave between each meal the bigger the health benefits will be.

Fresh ingredients are the way to go

This form of fasting isn't only good for your waist size it's also good for your wallet. Eating fresh, seasonal produce is not only the healthiest way to go it also provides excellent value. Pick up what's cheap and fresh at your local store. Those overripe red tomatoes will taste amazing when you roast them with herbs and balsamic vinegar. During the winter months, root vegetables like butternut squash and parsnip are tasty options in soup or roasted alone and served with some low-fat feta. You can take some halved peppers and stuff them with cream cheese, tuna, and vegetables before throwing them on the grill. The possibilities are nearly endless.

Fast low-calorie food swaps:

• Swap out your normal cappuccino for a black Americano.

• Swap out bananas for frozen or fresh berries in yogurt.

• Swap out higher fatty hard cheeses for lower-fat feta, ricotta, or reduced fat cream cheese.

• Swap out flans or quiches for an omelette.

• Swap out rice for cauliflower rice.

3. Eat-Stop-Eat

Eat-Stop-Eat form of fasting involves a 24-hour fast, either 1 or 2 times each week. This method was made popular by Brad Pilon a fitness expert and has caught on in popularity over the past few years. By fasting from dinner time on one day until dinner time on the next day you've completed a 24-hour fast. For example, finishing dinner at 8pm on Tuesday and not eating again until 8 pm on Wednesday. The time that you fast from doesn't matter. It can be from breakfast to breakfast, lunch to lunch or from midnight on one day until midnight the following day. However you slice it, the end result remains the same.

During the fasting period, you're allowed to drink coffee, water, and other beverages containing zero calories. You are not allowed to eat solid foods of any kind. During your normal eating periods, you can resume how you would normally eat although if you're looking to lose weight I would suggest switching to a low-fat diet. Many people struggle in the beginning going for 24 hours straight without eating. It's perfectly fine to begin with smaller intervals of 14 to 16 hours and slowly work your way up to a full 24-hour fasting period. I started out at 16 hours for the first few weeks and found it to be a good way to ease into the longer periods of fasting.

4. Alternate-Day Fasting

Alternate-Day Fasting is a form of Intermittent Fasting that requires you to fast on every other day of the week. There are a few different versions of this type of fast. Some of them allow you to consume 500 calories during your fasting days. A full fast every other day is extreme, so I wouldn't recommend this for anyone new to fasting.

Using this method, you will be probably be going to bed hungry a few times each week. In the long run, this version of fasting is probably not the most sustainable. I tried this for a few weeks and was miserable towards the end. It was definitely not for me and not something I would recommend considering the other equally effective alternatives.

5. The Warrior Diet

The Warrior Diet involves fasting during the daytime and eating a large meal at night. This form of Intermittent Fasting was made popular by Ori Hofmekler a fitness expert. This fasting diet involves eating a small amount of vegetables and raw fruits during the daytime, then eating one large meal at night. You're basically "fasting" all day and "feasting" at night within a small 4-hour eating period. The Warrior Diet is one of the first popular "diets" that include a form of Intermittent Fasting. This type of diet also places an emphasis on food choices that are very similar to someone following a Paleo Diet as it focuses on unprocessed whole foods that resemble what they looked like when found in nature.

6. Spontaneous Meal Skipping

This form of fasting is all about skipping meals when it is convenient. On this fast, you don't actually follow any type of structured Intermittent Fasting plan. You simply fast from time to time, skip a meal when you're not feeling hungry or are too busy to actually cook and sit down to eat. It is a common myth that we need to eat every couple of hours or we'll go into "starvation mode" and begin to lose muscle. Our bodies are well equipped to handle periods of long famine, let alone missing a few meals here and there. These shorter fasts are great because with a little practice you'll begin to find ways to fit them in all the time. This is also great for people just trying to maintain their current health or lose a few pounds.

Skipping a few meals when you feel like it is basically a form of spontaneous fasting. Just be sure to have healthy foods at your other meals. Skipping meals is pointless if you just gorge yourself with junk food the next time you eat. I know a ton of people who have gotten wonderful results with this method. I find that it is the best way to give Intermittent Fasting a try without diving in head first. It will allow you to gradually learn how your body responds to fasting and whether or not you deem it's something that's right for you.

Chapter Three: 20+ Intermittent Fasting Tips & Tricks

1. This one is obvious. Drink plenty of water. A good rule is 8 cups or 64 ounces day.

2. Integrate this diet into your daily lifestyle. Begin by slowly delaying breakfast. Doing this will allow you to ease it into your life until you get to a time you can live with. My time is about 1 pm.

3. Drink water when you get up in the morning. Often when we feel hungry in the morning, it's because we haven't had a drink of water for the past 8 hours. A healthy weight loss habit to follow is to drink 2 cups of water shortly after waking up.

4. Drink tea and coffee to help keep your appetite in check. Caffeine is a known natural appetite suppressant. Avoid drinking about 10 hours before you go to bed.

5. Make the diet flexible for you. Creating your own schedule allows you to have Intermittent Fasting work for you instead of you being a slave to it. This diet plan was meant to give you options.

6. Get your most productive work done during the morning. This will help keep your mind occupied and off of food.

7. Take Vitamin B. It helps you cope with stress and maintain healthy energy levels.

8. Play around with the "timing" of your eating schedule. It's important to follow a structured program for the first 2 to 3 weeks before going off and experimenting on your own. You need to follow a structured program at first and then you can play around with your fasting times and determine what schedule best suits your needs.

9. Stick to this diet for at least 3 weeks before making a final determination on if this diet is right for you. Your body needs this time to adapt.

10. Don't announce to other people that you're currently fasting. Even though this diet is beginning to gain more mainstream recognition, there are still a ton of folks who don't get the benefits of Intermittent Fasting. You don't need additional pressure or negativity putting you in the wrong mindset.

11. Live life to the fullest. Go crazy when you want. This diet is all about lifestyle and freedom. Just understand you'll need to adjust your calorie intake during the following day or two.

12. If you decide to follow a 24-hour Alternate Day Fast (ADF) keep them to only 2 times per week.

13. Workout with weights. There is less point of fasting if you don't plan to workout using weights. You need to build your muscle mass to take full advantage of all the benefits that come from Intermittent Fasting.

14. Your first meal will set the tone for your remaining meals that day. Keep your first meal each day as healthy as you can because it will keep you on track for your following meals. This tip made sticking to my diet a breeze. Conversely, whenever I ate poorly during my initial daily meal I continued to struggle throughout the rest of the day. Set yourself up for success from the get-go.

15. Exercise but don't feel the need to overdo it. I recommend combining an exercise routine with IF to see the optimal results. That being said, I know many who burn themselves out by hitting their workouts too hard. These people tend to give up on the diet altogether or struggle to eat healthily.

16. Have a lot of protein in each meal. More protein leads to better appetite control and will help to burn fat and build muscle.

17. Don't sit around your house. There is way too much temptation waiting for you at home. Get creative and do something active while you begin your IF.

18. Expect there to be peaks and valleys. They are a normal part of life. By keeping an open mind and not freaking out during "down" periods you'll figure out how to have more "ups."

19. Don't use IF as a reason to eat a lot of junk food. All calories are not created equally. 100 calories of chocolate are not the same as 100 calories of vegetables. When you find yourself about to cheat take a few minutes and think through what you're doing. Eat whole foods and keep carbs to your post workout window. Fill up with vegetables and include plenty of protein in each meal.

20. Understand what else is happening in your life at the time. IF is a nutrition style that will work. However, it only "works" when it's intermittent, flexible, and part of your daily routine. Intermittent Fasting shouldn't feel like an obligation or a punishment. If this type of diet is doing more harm than good to your psychological well-being, it might not be right for you. The whole point is to get healthier and decrease stress levels.

21. When starting IF stay busy with meaningful work. I tend to get my best work done while I'm on an empty stomach.

22. Respect the cues your body gives you. Paying attention to these cues is extremely important. These cues can include big changes in your appetite and hunger including food cravings, energy levels, sleep quality, mood control, athletic performance, emotional health, physical health, and appearance.

23. Know yourself. Observe your personal experiences carefully. When it comes to your well-being pretend you're a scientist. Begin IF, gather data, gain new insights, and come up with conclusions that you can use to help decide future action. Always do what's best for you.

24. When starting IF stay busy with meaningful work. I tend to get my best work done while I'm on an empty stomach.

25. Consider where the source of your hunger stems from. A feeling of hunger is often brought on by other outside stimuli that don't include actual hunger. Some examples include, stress, dehydration, anxiety, and feelings of sadness. Once you've determined the reason you're hungry you'll be better equipped to deal with that hunger.

Chapter Four: Intermittent Fasting Resources, Apps, & Books

Intermittent Fasting Resource Guide

In this section, I will go over my top Intermittent Fasting resources. There's a ton of information on the subject. If you have any lingering questions, I'd be surprised if you couldn't find it using one of the resources below.

Eat, Fast & Live Longer - Here is a link to an informative 1-hour documentary that I watched when first starting out.

https://www.youtube.com/watch?v=Ihhj_VSKiTs

Intermittent Fasting for Beginners - Great site with a lot of good information. Also includes videos, recipes, and other helpful resources to help you get started.

https://www.dietdoctor.com/intermittent-fasting

Intermittent Fasting for Women - Good collection of articles and resources specifically geared towards women.

http://runholy.com/intermittent-fasting-resources-for-women/

Recipe Calorie Counter - If you're counting calories this site is great. You can type in a recipe and it spits out the nutrition information. It's fast and it's free.

https://www.verywell.com/recipe-nutrition-analyzer-4129594

The 5:2 Fast Diet Website - Instructions for how to get started. Offers some helpful tools and a good forum to get answers to any questions that might come up.

https://thefastdiet.co.uk/

Intermittent Fasting App Guide

In this section, I'm going to go over all my favorite apps related to Intermittent Fasting. These are apps that I've used at least one time. I'm sure there are many others I may have missed but this section will give you a small idea of the different types of apps available to you. I recommend trying a few out and keeping the ones that suit your particular needs.

5:2 Fast Diet Tracker - Free app available only on Android. Great app specific to people following a 5:2 fast. Lots of helpful features and tracking.

5:2 Fasting Diet Recipes - Costs $1.99. Available on the iOS only. Comes with over 80 calories counted recipes broken down into different sections so what you want is easy to find. Separated into 100, 200, and 300 calories sections.

Fasting Secret - Available on the iOS only. Free basic version along with $1.99 pro upgrade. Works perfectly with intermittent, 5:2, 16:8, and alternate day fasting diet plans. One of my personal favorites.

IF Diet - Free app available only iOS. Offers a lot of customizable features to fit any type of intermittent diet. Includes weight manager, fasting countdown, and calorie intake calculator.

Intermittent Fasting - Free app available only on Android. Has a nice set of features that are simple to navigate.

MyFast Intermittent Fasting - Free app available only on Android. Not my personal favorite but a reliable fasting app.

Vora Fasting Tracker - Free app available only on Android. Vora is a cloud-based fasting tracker that allows you to create, edit, and delete your fasts. View your last 7 fasts in a beautiful chart that shows if you're reaching your fasting target.

Zero Fasting Tracker - Free app available only on iOS. Zero is a simple fasting tracker used for intermittent, circadian rhythm, and custom fasting. Great features and easy to use.

Intermittent Fasting Book Guide

Here are some of my favorite books on Intermittent Fasting. I've read a bunch on this subject over the years and these are some of the books that made a lasting impression and got me started in the right direction when I was a newbie.

1. **The 8-Hour Diet** by David Zinczenko

2. **The Warrior Diet** by Ori Hofmekler

3. **The FastDiet** by Michael Mosley

4. **The IF Diet** by Robert Skinner

Chapter Five: Intermittent Fasting Breakfast Recipes

In this section, I will share with you 10+ Intermittent Fasting breakfast recipes you can prepare yourself. I'll include both beginner recipes and some advanced recipes. That way no matter what your skill level in the kitchen you'll be able to create a healthy low-calorie meal.

Summer Vegetable Omelette with Salsa (Serves 2)

Ingredients:

Omelette:

4 Eggs

2 cups of 1% Milk or Skim Milk

Pepper

Salt

Filling:

2 3/4 ounces of Fine Asparagus Spears

3 1/2 ounces of Cherry Tomatoes (Whole)

3 1/2 ounces of Mushrooms (Thickly Sliced)

3 1/2 ounces of Baby Corn

Serve:

3 1/2 ounces of Fresh Salsa

Directions:

1. Beat your eggs with your milk, and season with some pepper and salt.

2. Slice your baby sweetcorn in half, and add with your asparagus to a large-sized frying pan. Saute for approximately 5 minutes.

3. Add your mushrooms (thickly sliced) and cherry tomatoes (whole) to your frying pan.

4. Meanwhile, divide your egg mixture between 2 smaller-sized omelette pans and cook over a medium heat. Once the bottom layer of your egg has solidified enough to hold its shape, flip your omelette to cook the other side.

5. Once your egg is fully cooked, divide your filling between the 2 omelettes, and add a scoop of fresh salsa.

6. Serve and Enjoy!

Coconut Flour Porridge Breakfast Cereal (Serves 1)

Ingredients:

2 tablespoons of Coconut Flour

1 Large Egg (Beaten)

2 tablespoons of Golden Flax Meal

2 teaspoons of Butter

3/4 cup of Water

1 tablespoon of Sukrin Gold

1 tablespoon of Heavy Cream

Salt

Directions:

1.Place your coconut flour, golden flax meal, salt, and water into a small-sized pot over medium high heat. When it begins to simmer, turn it down to medium and whisk until it begins to thicken.

2. Remove your coconut flour porridge from the heat and add the beaten egg, little by little, while whisking continuously. Place back on the heat and continue to whisk until the porridge thickens.

3. Remove from the heat and continue to whisk for approximately 30 seconds before adding your butter, cream, and sweetener.

4. Garnish with your favorite toppings.

5. Serve and Enjoy!

Fennel & Ginger Grain Free Granola (Serves 20)

Ingredients:

4 cups of Shredded Coconut (Unsweetened)

1 cup of Sunflower Seeds

1 cup of Pumpkin Seeds

2 tablespoons of Dried Fennel Seeds

2 tablespoons of Ground Ginger

2 tablespoons of Ground Cardamom

5 tablespoons of Granulated Sweetener

1/4 cup of Coconut Oil (Melted)

Directions:

1. Place all your ingredients in a large-side roasting dish.

2. Mix together with a large-sized spoon.

3. Bake in your oven at 350 degrees for 20 minutes but you must turn the mixture every 3 to 4 minutes.

4. Once the entire grain free granola is browned and baked, remove from your oven and allow it to cool completely before placing in your storage jars.

5. Serve and Enjoy!

Low-Carb Cereal (Serves 15)

Ingredients:

1 cup of Sunflower Seeds

1 cup of Pumpkin Seeds

1 cup Unsweetened Flaked Coconut

1 cup of Sliced Almonds

2 teaspoons of Cinnamon

1/2 cup of Pecans

1/2 cup of Hemp Hearts

1/4 teaspoon of Vanilla Stevia Drops

1/2 teaspoon of Vanilla Extract

Directions:

1. In your large-sized bowl, stir together all of your ingredients until well combined.

2. Lay out on your rimmed baking pan and bake at 350 degrees for approximately 7 to 8 minutes.

3. Allow it to cool. Store in an air tight container.

4. Serve and Enjoy!

Low-Carb Waffles (Serves 1)

Ingredients:

3 Egg Whites

2 tablespoons of Coconut Flour

1/2 teaspoon of Baking Powder

2 tablespoons of Unsweetened Almond Milk

1 packet of Stevia

Directions:

1. Whip 2 of your egg whites to stiff peaks.

2. Once you have stiff peaks, stir in your coconut flour, milk, stevia, baking powder, sweetener, and 1 egg white.

3. Heat up your waffle iron to the highest temperature, and grease or spray it with your nonstick spray. Pour in your batter.

4. Cook in your waffle iron until brown. Should take approximately 3 to 4 minutes. Remove and add any desired toppings.

5. Serve and Enjoy!

Spinach, Goat Cheese, & Chorizo Omelette (Serves 2)

Ingredients:

4 ounces of Chorizo Sausage

4 Eggs

1/2 tablespoon of Butter

1 tablespoon of Water

2 cups of Baby Spinach Leaves

2 ounces of Crumbled Fresh Goat Cheese

1/4 cup of Salsa Verde (Optional)

Sliced Avocado (Optional)

Directions:

1. Remove your chorizo from the casing and fry in your medium saute pan until fully cooked.

2. Meanwhile, beat your eggs and water in a small-sized bowl.

3. Take your chorizo out of your pan with a slotted spoon and set to the side. Wipe the pan of any remaining grease with a clean paper towel.

4. Melt your butter in the same pan over a low heat. Add your beaten eggs to the pan, then put the Chorizo, spinach, and crumbled goat cheese on half your egg mixture. Cook on a low heat for 3 minutes until slightly firm, then fold the empty side over the side with the filling on it.

5. Cover your pan with foil or a pot cover and leave on a low heat for another few minutes until your eggs are cooked through. If your bottom is browning too quickly, turn your stove off and leave your pan covered for up to 10 minutes and the residual heat should "bake" it until the center is fully cooked.

6. Add avocado slices and salsa verde if desired.

7. Serve and Enjoy!

Veggie Breakfast Burritos (Serves 4)

Ingredients:

4 Eggs

6 Chestnut Mushrooms

2 tablespoons of Sunflower Oil

1 Potato (Baked, Boiled, or Steamed)

1 Red Onion

3 1/2 ounces of Cheese

1 Sweet Red Pepper

2 Vegetarian Sausages

4 Large Tortilla Wraps

Directions:

1. Chop your mushrooms, pepper, onion, and potato into smaller-sized pieces.

2. Heat 2 teaspoons of your oil in a large-sized frying pan and fry your vegetables until soft.

3. Heat another 1 teaspoon of oil and fry your sausages according to the packet instructions. Set to the side.

4. Add your remaining oil to your pan, bring up to temperature and add your eggs. Scramble lightly as they cook.

5. Chop your cooled sausages into chunks and grate your cheese.

6. Gently warm your tortillas. A few seconds in the microwave should be more than enough.

7. Divide your ingredients equally between the 4 tortillas.

8. Arrange the filling in a line down the middle of your tortilla, leaving some room clear at each end of the line, then fold one edge of your tortilla along the length of the filling. Turn in the two adjacent edge and continue to roll in the direction of your first fold.

9. When you're ready to eat them, microwave your burritos to reheat the fillings. I found about 1 minute was perfect to warm them from the fridge.

10. Serve and Enjoy!

Eggs & Bacon w/ A Twist (Serves 6)

<u>Ingredients:</u>

6 Hard-Cooked Organic Extra Large Eggs

3 1/2 ounces of Cream Cheese

12 slices of Organic Bacon

1/4 teaspoon of Dried Organic Thyme

<u>Directions:</u>

1. Preheat your oven to 400 degrees.

2. Prepare your cream cheese filling: Combine your cream cheese and thyme in a small-sized bowl and mix with your spoon until well mixed. Cover and set to the side.

3. Peel your eggs and cut them lengthwise with a sharp knife.

4. Remove your yolks.

5. Fill the 6 egg white halves with your cream cheese filling. Cover with your remaining 6 egg white halves.

6. Take 2 bacon slices per filled egg and wrap your eggs tightly in your bacon slices.

7. Place your wrapped eggs in a shallow ceramic or glass baking dish and bake for approximately 30 minutes.

8. Remove from your oven.

9. Serve and Enjoy!

Baked Eggs w/ Spinach & Yogurt (Serves 4)

Ingredients:

4 Large Eggs

2/3 cup of Plain Greek-Style Yogurt

1/4 teaspoon of Crushed Red Pepper Flakes

2 tablespoons of Unsalted Butter

2 tablespoons of Olive Oil

2 tablespoons of Chopped Scallion (White & Pale-Green Parts Only)

3 tablespoons of Chopped Leek (White & Pale-Green Parts Only)

1 teaspoon of Fresh Lemon Juice

10 cups of Fresh Spinach

1 Garlic Clove (Halved)

1 teaspoon of Chopped Fresh Oregano

Kosher Salt

<u>Directions:</u>

1. Mix your garlic, yogurt, and a pinch of salt in your small-sized bowl. Set to the side.

2. Preheat your oven to 300 degrees. Melt 1 tablespoon of butter with your oil in a large-sized heavy skillet over a medium heat. Add your scallion and leek and reduce the heat to low. Cook until soft, approximately 10 minutes. Add your spinach and lemon juice. Season with salt. Increase the heat to a medium-high and cook, turning frequently, until wilted. Should take approximately 4 to 5 minutes.

3. Transfer your spinach mixture to a 10-inch skillet, leaving any of the excess liquid behind. If you're using 2 smaller-sized skillets, divide your spinach mixture equally between the skillets. Make 4 deep indentations in the center of your spinach in the larger-sized skillet or 2 indentations in each small-sized skillet. Carefully break 1 egg into each hollow, taking care to keep the yolks intact. Bake until your egg whites are set. Should take approximately 10 to 15 minutes.

4. Melt your remaining 1 tablespoon of butter in a small-sized saucepan over a medium-low heat. Add your crushed red pepper flakes and a pinch of salt and cook until your butter begins to foam and browned bits form at bottom of your pan. Should take approximately 1 to 2 minutes. Add your oregano and cook for an additional 30 seconds.

5. Remove your garlic halves from the yogurt and discard. Spoon your yogurt over the spinach and eggs. Drizzle with your spiced butter.

6. Serve and Enjoy!

Ham & Cheese Crepes (Serves 4)

Ingredients:

Crepes:

6 Large Eggs

6 ounces of Cream Cheese (Softened)

1 1/2 tablespoons of Coconut Flour

1/3 cup of Grated Parmesan Cheese

1 teaspoon of Erythritol

1/8 teaspoon of Xanthan Gum

1 tablespoon of Melted Butter

Ham & Swiss Filling:

6 ounces of Swiss Cheese (Shaved or Grated)

3 ounces of Black Forest Ham

Directions:

1. Place your eggs, Parmesan cheese, cream cheese, and erythritol in your blender. Blend on low until your ingredients are well combined. With your blender running, sprinkle your coconut flour and the xanthan gum over the batter and continue blending until thick, scraping the sides down at least one time. Finish with the blender on a medium speed for a couple seconds. Allow the batter to sit for approximately 10 minutes.

2. Place a non-stick pan over a medium heat. Lightly brush your pan with butter. Lightly brush your spatula.

3. Stir your batter. Pour your batter into a 1/4 cup measure and then into the middle of your pan. Resist the urge to scrape the measuring cup out with your finger. Grasp the pan by the handle and begin tilting it in a circular motion to help spread your batter into a circle. It won't be perfect and that's fine.

4. Let your crepe cook for about 1 1/2 minutes or until the top of your crepe looks dull and the edge begins to brown. Gently work the spatula under the edge of your crepe by shimmying it and lift the edge. With the fingers of your other hand, grasp the crepe gently and lift it while sliding your spatula under the crepe further. Flip your crepe and allow it to cook for approximately 15 to 20 seconds.

5. Remove your crepe to the plate and begin the process again making sure to lightly butter your pan and the spatula after each crepe. Stack your crepes one on top of the other. Allow it to cool and refrigerate or use right away.

6. Pre-heat your oven to 175 degrees. Heat a non-stick pan over a medium to a medium-low heat. When hot, put one crepe in the center of the pan and add about 1/4 cup of grated cheese. Place your ham on one side of the crepe. Cook until the cheese has begun to melt. Should take about 1 minute. Fold the side of your crepe without the ham over the ham forming a half circle. Then fold in half making a quarter circle. Place the filled crepe on the platter and into the warm oven. Continue until all of your crepes have been filled.

7. Serve and Enjoy!

Bacon Pancakes (Serves 2)

Ingredients:

6 slices of Bacon

3 Egg Whites

1/4 cup of Coconut Flour

1 tablespoon of Purified Granular Gelatin

2 tablespoons Unsalted Butter (Melted)

2 tablespoons of Finely Chopped Chives

1/2 cup of Water

Directions:

1. Cook your bacon in your frying pan over a medium heat. Leave your bacon fat in your pan. Crumble or finely chop your bacon and set to the side.

2. Whisk your egg whites into soft peaks Set to the side.

3. In your large-sized bowl mix together the coconut flour, butter, gelatin, chives, and bacon. Add your water and mix well then gently fold in your egg whites until combined. The batter will be thick and lumpy.

4. Re-heat your bacon fat in the frying pan over a medium heat. Scoop about 2 tablespoons of batter into your pan, gently smoothing the batter out with a spoon to form small-sized pancakes.

5. Cook for approximately 3 minutes on each side.

6. Serve and Enjoy!

Breakfast Chili (Serves 8)

Ingredients:

Chili:

2 pounds of Ground Grass Fed Beef

1 pound of Spicy Italian Sausage

1/2 Chopped Yellow Onion

4 cups of Tomato Sauce

2 slices of Bacon

3 stalks of Chopped Celery

1 Red Bell Pepper (Seeded & Chopped)

1 Green Bell Pepper (Seeded & Chopped)

2 Green Chile Peppers (Seeded & Chopped)

1/4 cup of Chili Powder

1 cup of Organic Beef Broth

1 tablespoon of Minced Garlic

1 teaspoon of Ground Black Pepper

3 tablespoons of Fresh Oregano

1 teaspoon of Celtic Sea Salt

2 teaspoons of Ground Cumin

1 teaspoon of Cayenne Pepper

3 tablespoons of Fresh Basil

1 teaspoon of Paprika

Toppings:

Fried Eggs

Avocado (Cubed)

Bacon (Fried & Crumbled)

Bread Bowl:

3 Eggs

1/2 teaspoon of Cream of Tartar

1/4 cup of Unflavored Egg White

3 ounces of Organic Sour Cream

Directions:

1. Heat your large-sized stock pot over a medium-high heat. Crumble your ground chuck, bacon and sausage into your hot pan, and cook until evenly browned. Drain off any excess grease. Pour in your tomato sauce. Add your onion, celery, green, chile peppers, red bell peppers, and broth. Season with your chili powder, oregano, garlic, basil, cumin, pepper, cayenne, salt, and paprika. Stir to blend, then cover and simmer over a low heat for approximately 2 hours, stirring occasionally. After 2 hours, taste, and adjust your salt, pepper, and chili powder if necessary. The longer your chili simmers, the better it will begin to taste. Remove from heat. Top with a fried egg, avocado and bacon pieces.

2. To make your bread bowl: Preheat your oven to 350 degrees. Separate your eggs (reserve the yolks). In a clean and dry bowl, whip your egg whites and cream of tartar until stiff. Then add the protein powder until smooth. Using your spatula, gradually fold your sour cream into the white mixture, being careful not to break down the whites. Grease your muffin tins and spoon your mixture into the pan (forming a dip in the middle), making 12 medium-sized bowls or 24 mini bowls. Bake at 350 degrees for approximately 12 to 15 minutes. You may need to put the center down once they come out so you can fill it with chili.

3. Serve and Enjoy!

Salmon & Avocado Breakfast (Serves 1)

Ingredients:

2 ounces of Wild Smoked Salmon

1 Ripe Organic Avocado

2 tablespoons of Organic Extra Virgin Olive Oil

1 ounces of Soft Goat Cheese

1 Lemon (Juiced)

Celtic Sea Salt

Directions:

1. Cut your avocado in two and remove the seed.

2. In your small food processor, mix the rest of your ingredients until coarsely chopped.

3. Place the resulting cream inside your avocado.

4. Serve and Enjoy!

Snickerdoodle Mug Cake (Serves 2)

Ingredients:

2 teaspoons of Swerve Sweetener (For Small Bowl)

2 tablespoons of Swerve Sweetener (For Medium Bowl)

1/2 teaspoon of Ground Cinnamon

2/3 cup of Almond Flour

1 Large Egg

1 teaspoon of Baking Powder

1/4 teaspoon of Cinnamon

1/8 teaspoon of Cream of Tartar

2 tablespoons of Melted Butter

1/4 teaspoon of Vanilla Extract

2 tablespoons of Water

Pinch of Salt

Directions:

1. In your small-sized bowl, whisk together the sweetener and cinnamon. Set to the side.

2. In your medium-sized bowl, whisk together your almond flour, baking powder, sweetener, salt, cinnamon, and cream of tartar.

3. Add your egg, butter, water, and vanilla extract and stir until well combined.

4. Divide half your batter between two coffee mugs. Sprinkle with half of the topping mixture. Divide remaining batter between mugs and sprinkle with the remaining topping mixture.

5. Cook on high in microwave for 1 minute, until puffed and just barely cooked through.

6. Add cream or milk if desired.

7. Serve and Enjoy!

Chapter Six: Intermittent Fasting Lunch Recipes

In this section, I will share with you 10+ Intermittent Fasting lunch recipes you can prepare yourself. I'll include both beginner recipes and some advanced recipes. That way no matter what your skill level in the kitchen you'll be able to create a healthy low-calorie meal.

Smoked Salmon Chowder (Serves 8)

Ingredients:

1 pound of Potatoes (Peeled & Cubed)

8 ounces of Smoked Salmon (Cut Into 1/2-Inch Pieces)

2 tablespoons of Butter

1 tablespoon of Olive Oil

2 cloves of Chopped Garlic

1 cup of Chopped Onion

1/2 cup of All-Purpose Flour

1/2 teaspoon of Paprika

1/2 cup of Chopped Celery

6 cups of Chicken Broth

1/4 teaspoon of Hot Sauce

1 teaspoon of Dried Tarragon

1 teaspoon of Dried Dill Weed

1 teaspoon of Ground Black Pepper

1 teaspoon of Dried Thyme

1 tablespoon of Fresh Lemon Juice

1/4 cup of White Wine

1 teaspoon of Salt

1 cup Half and Half

<u>Directions:</u>

1. In your large-sized stock pot over a medium-high heat, combine your butter, onion, olive oil, garlic, and celery. Cook approximately 8 to 10 minutes, or until your onions are transparent. Sprinkle flour over the mixture and stir well to make a dry roux. Gradually add your chicken broth and stir until slightly thickened. Stir in your potatoes, dill, thyme, tarragon, and paprika. Reduce heat to a medium, cover, and simmer for approximately 15 minutes.

2. Stir in your salmon, lemon juice, wine, hot sauce, pepper, and salt. Simmer over a low heat, uncovered for approximately 10 minutes.

3. Mix in your half-and-half and continue to simmer for approximately 30 minutes, stirring occasionally. Do not let your chowder boil after adding the half-and-half.

4. Serve and Enjoy!

BBQ Chicken Cobb Salad (Serves 4)

<u>Ingredients:</u>

<u>*Salad:*</u>

2 Boneless, Skinless Thin-Sliced Chicken Breasts

4 slices of Bacon (Diced)

3 tablespoons of BBQ Sauce

6 cups of Chopped Romaine Lettuce

2 Large Eggs

2 Roma Tomatoes (Diced)

1 cup of Canned Corn Kernels (Drained)

1 Avocado (Halved, Seeded, Peeled & Diced)

1 cup of Canned Black Beans (Drained & Rinsed)

Kosher Salt

Freshly Ground Black Pepper

<u>*Buttermilk Ranch Dressing:*</u>

1/4 cup of Plain Greek Yogurt

1/2 cup of Buttermilk

1/4 cup of Sour Cream

1/4 teaspoon of Garlic Powder

1/2 teaspoon of Dried Dill

1/2 teaspoon of Dried Parsley

Kosher Salt

Freshly Ground Black Pepper

Directions:

1. To make your buttermilk ranch dressing, whisk together your buttermilk, Greek yogurt, dill, sour cream, garlic powder, parsley, salt, and pepper in a small-sized bowl. Set to the side.

2. Heat your large-sized skillet over a medium high heat. Add your bacon and cook until brown and crispy. Should take approximately 6 to 8 minutes. Transfer to your paper towel-lined plate. Set to the side.

3. Season your chicken breasts with salt and pepper. Add to skillet and cook, flipping once, until cooked through. Should take approximately 3 to 4 minutes per side. Allow it to cool before dicing into bite-size pieces.

4. In your medium-sized bowl, add your chicken and BBQ sauce. Gently toss to combine. Set to the side.

5. Place your eggs in a large-sized saucepan and cover with cold water by 1-inch. Bring to a boil and cook for approximately 1 minute. Cover your eggs with a tight-fitting lid and remove from the heat. Set to the side for approximately 8 to 10 minutes. Drain well and allow it to cool before peeling and dicing.

6. To assemble your salad, place your romaine lettuce in a large-sized bowl. Top with your arranged rows of bacon, eggs, BBQ chicken, avocado, tomatoes, beans, and corn.

7. Add your buttermilk ranch dressing as desired.

8. Serve and Enjoy!

California Turkey & Bacon Lettuce Wraps w/ Basil-Mayo (Serves 2)

Ingredients:

1 head of Iceberg Lettuce

4 slices of Gluten-Free Deli Turkey

4 slices of Gluten-Free Bacon (Cooked)

1 Avocado (Thinly Sliced)

1 Roma Tomato (Thinly Sliced)

Basil-Mayo:

1/2 cup of Gluten-Free Mayonnaise

6 large of Basil Leaves (Torn)

1 teaspoon of Lemon Juice

1 Chopped Garlic Clove

Salt

Pepper

<u>Directions:</u>

1. For your basil-mayo combine the ingredients in your small food processor then process until smooth.

2. Lay out 2 large lettuce leaves then layer on 1 slice of turkey and slather with your Basil-Mayo. Layer on the second slice of your turkey followed by your bacon, and a couple slices of both tomato and avocado. Lightly season with salt and pepper then fold the bottom up, the sides in, and roll it up like a burrito. Slice in half.

3. Serve and Enjoy!

Acorn Squash w/ Sesame Greens (Serves 2)

<u>Ingredients:</u>

1 Acorn Squash

1 teaspoon of Olive Oil

3 1/2 ounces of Kale

3 1/2 ounces of Cabbage

5 Large Garlic Cloves

2 tablespoons of Sesame Seeds

1 tablespoon of Soy Sauce

1 tablespoon of Toasted Sesame Oil

<u>Directions:</u>

1. Preheat your oven to 390 degrees.

2. Scrub the skin of the squash, then slice in half and scrape out any seeds.

3. Brush your squash flesh with olive oil. Bake for approximately 25 minutes until soft.

4. Finely shred your kale and cabbage.

5. In your large-sized frying pan, warm your cabbage and kale over a low heat with your sesame seeds. Stir frequently to prevent sticking.

6. After about 15 minutes, once your vegetables have started to wilt, crush and add your garlic. Toss with the soy sauce and sesame oil.

7. Heap your wilted greens in the squash.

8. Serve and Enjoy!

Warm Asparagus & Mushroom Salad (Serves 1)

Ingredients:

12 Asparagus Spears

8 Medium Chestnut Mushrooms

1 Spring Green Onion

8 Walnut Halves

1 teaspoon of Soy Sauce

1 teaspoon of Shaoxing Rice Wine

Handful of Fresh Coriander

Directions:

1. Rinse, trim, and chop your vegetables. Quarter the mushrooms, cut your asparagus into 3 to 4 pieces, and finely slice your spring onion.

2. In your frying pan, sauté your asparagus and mushroom over a medium heat.

3. Once your vegetables begin to soften, add your spring onion, soy sauce, and rice wine to your pan, and continue to sauté until your spring onions are cooked and the liquid has reduced.

4. Meanwhile, heat your separate frying pan to a high temperature, and toast your walnuts until they are golden brown and the oils are beginning to emerge.

5. Toss your walnuts together with your asparagus mixture. Add the fresh coriander.

6. Serve and Enjoy!

Asparagus & Smoked Salmon Salad (Serves 8)

Ingredients:

1/4 pound of Smoked Salmon (Cut Into 1-Inch Chunks)

1 pound of Fresh Asparagus (Trimmed & Cut Into 1-Inch Pieces)

1/2 cup of Pecans (Broken Into Pieces)

1/2 cup of Frozen Green Peas (Thawed)

2 heads of Red Leaf Lettuce (Rinsed & Torn)

1/4 cup of Olive Oil

1 teaspoon of Dijon Mustard

2 tablespoons of Lemon Juice

1/2 teaspoon of Salt

Directions:

1. Bring your pot of water to a boil. Place your asparagus in your pot. Cook for approximately 5 minutes until tender. Drain and set to the side.

2. Place your pecans in a skillet over a medium heat. Cook approximately 5 minutes, stirring frequently, until lightly toasted.

3. In your large-sized bowl, toss together your pecans, asparagus, red leaf lettuce, salmon, and peas.

4. In your separate bowl, mix your olive oil, Dijon mustard, lemon juice, salt, and pepper. Toss with your salad.

5. Serve and Enjoy!

Chickpea & Salmon Salad (Serves 6)

<u>Ingredients:</u>

3 cans of Salmon (Drained)

2 cans of Chickpeas (Rinsed & Drained)

5 stalks of Celery (Thinly Sliced)

2 Bell Peppers (Thinly Sliced)

2 cloves of Garlic (Finely Minced)

3 Shallots (Finely Minced)

1/2 cup of Olive Oil

1 Large Cucumber (Halved & Sliced)

1 Lemon (Juiced & Zested)

1 pint of Halved Tomatoes

1 tablespoon of Red Wine Vinegar

1 teaspoon of Fresh or Dried Dill

1/2 teaspoon of Freshly Ground Black Pepper

1/2 teaspoon of Ground Cumin

1/2 teaspoon of Smoked Paprika

1/2 teaspoon of Crushed Red Pepper Flakes

1 teaspoon of Kosher Salt

Directions:

1. Finely mince and chop your celery, garlic, shallots, bell peppers, cucumber, and tomatoes. Add them to a large-sized bowl with your chickpeas. Toss together with your olive oil, lemon juice and zest, red wine vinegar, salt, dill, cumin, black pepper, paprika, and crushed red pepper flakes.

2. Drain your cans of salmon and add them to your bowl. Toss to combine. Allow the salad to sit for an hour or so in the refrigerator, taste, adjust seasonings as needed.

3. Serve and Enjoy!

Smoked Salmon Pitta Pizza (Serves 1)

Ingredients:

1 White Pitta Bread

1 ounce of Smoked Salmon Slices

1 tablespoon of Low Fat Cream Cheese Chive and Onion

1 teaspoon of Drained Capers

1/4 Red Onion (Peeled & Finely Diced)

1 1/2 ounces of Lettuce Leaves

1 Lemon Wedge

Fresh or Dried Dill

Directions:

1. Preheat your oven to 350 degrees.

2. Spread your pitta bread with your low-fat cream cheese then top with your smoked salmon pieces. Scatter the red onion over the top and then the capers.

3. Bake for approximately 10 minutes, or until your pitta bread is golden and crispy around the edges.

4. Add your lemon wedge and fresh chopped dill as well as some fresh lettuce leaves.

5. Serve and Enjoy!

Barbacoa (Serves 12)

Ingredients:

3 pounds of Chuck Toast (Fat Trimmed & Cut Into 2-Inch Chunks)

4-ounce can of Chopped Green Chiles

2 Chipotles in Adobo Sauce (Chopped)

1 Small White Onion (Finely Chopped)

2 tablespoons of Apple Cider Vinegar

1/4 cup of Fresh Lime Juice

4 cloves of Minced Garlic

3 Bay Leaves

1 tablespoon of Dried Mexican Oregano

1 tablespoon of Ground Cumin

1/4 teaspoon of Ground Cloves

1/2 cup of Beef Stock

2 teaspoons of Salt

1 teaspoon of Black Pepper

<u>Directions:</u>

1. Combine all your ingredients in the bowl of your slow cooker. Toss gently to combine. Cover and cook on low for approximately 6 to 8 hours, or on high for approximately 3 to 4 hours, or until your beef is tender and falls apart easily when shredded with a fork.

2. Using two forks, shred your beef into bite-sized pieces inside of the slow cooker. Toss your beef with the juices, then cover and let the barbacoa beef soak up the juices for an extra 10 minutes. Remove your bay leaves. Use a pair of tongs or a slotted spoon to serve the barbacoa beef.

3. If not using immediately, refrigerate the barbacoa beef with its juices in a sealed container for up to 5 days. You can also freeze it for up to 3 months.

4. Serve and Enjoy!

Shawarma Chicken Bowls w/ Basil-Lemon Vinaigrette (Serves 4)

<u>Ingredients:</u>

<u>Chicken Shawarma:</u>

1 pound of Free-Range Organic Chicken Breast (Cut Into 3-inch Strips)

3 Minced Garlic Cloves

2 tablespoons of Olive Oil

1/2 teaspoon of Ground Cumin

3/4 teaspoon of Fine Grain Sea Salt

2 tablespoons of Lemon Juice

1 teaspoon of Curry Powder

1/4 teaspoon of Ground Coriander

<u>Salad:</u>

6 cups of Spring Greens

2 handfuls of Torn Fresh Basil Leaves

1 cup of Halved Cherry Tomatoes

1 Sliced Avocado

<u>*Basil-Lemon Vinaigrette:*</u>

2 handfuls of Fresh Basil Leaves

1 Smashed Garlic Clove

2 tablespoons of Fresh Lemon Juice

1/2 teaspoon of Fine Grain Sea Salt

5 tablespoons of Olive Oil

Directions:

1. In your bowl, whisk your olive oil, lemon juice, salt, garlic, cumin, curry powder, and coriander until well combined.

2. In a large Ziploc bag, combine your chicken strips and marinade.

3. Seal and marinate in your refrigerator for a minimum of 20 minutes (marinate overnight for fullest flavor.)

4. When you're ready to make the meal, heat your large-sized nonstick skillet over a medium-high heat.

5. Add your olive oil and your chicken. Cook until golden brown and cooked through. Should take approximately 6 to 8 minutes turning regularly, until the juices run clear.

6. In the meantime make your vinaigrette. In your food processor or small blender, process your basil, garlic, salt, and lemon juice until smooth. With the motor running, slowly add the oil. Blend until well combined. Set to the side.

7. To make your salads, add your greens in a large-sized bowl and toss them with a sprinkle of salt and pepper. Add your chicken on top along with the tomatoes, basil, and avocado.

8. Drizzle the bowl with your basil-lemon vinaigrette.

9. Serve and Enjoy!

Portobello & Halloumi Burgers (Serves 2)

<u>Ingredients:</u>

4 Portobello Mushroom Caps w/ Stems Removed

2 tablespoons of Olive Oil

3 1/2 tablespoons of Balsamic Vinegar

2 Thick Slices of Tomato

2 Thin Slices of Halloumi Cheese

1 handful of Basil Leaves

Sea Salt

Pepper

<u>**Directions:**</u>

1. Heat grill to a medium-high heat (about 450 degrees). Wash your mushroom caps and cry. In your shallow bowl, combine your balsamic vinegar and olive oil. Place your mushrooms gill side down in the mixture.

2. When your grill is hot, grill the mushrooms on the gill side first for approximately 5 minutes or until they start to sweat. Flip and grill approximately 2 to 3 minutes more. Add your halloumi to the grill and grill 2 minutes on each side over relatively high heat until grill marks form on the cheese and it becomes soft and pliable. Sprinkle your salt and pepper onto the tomato.

3. Assemble your "burger" with the mushroom as the bun, the halloumi cheese as the burger, the lightly salted tomato, and fresh basil leaves.

4. Serve and Enjoy!

Simple Spaghetti Squash

Ingredients:

1 Spaghetti Squash

3/4 cup of Toasted Hazelnuts

1 1/2 cups of Cooked Chickpeas

1 bunch of Kale

3 cloves of Garlic

Pinch of Crushed Chilies

Pecorino Romano (Hard Sheep's Milk Cheese)

Olive Oil

Sea Salt

Directions:

1. Preheat your oven to 400 degrees.

2. Prepare your spaghetti squash by cutting it in half lengthwise, removing your seeds, rubbing the inside of each half with a drizzle of olive oil, then seasoning with your salt and pepper. Place face down on a lined baking tray and place in your oven. Cook for approximately 45 minutes.

3. While your squash is baking, prepare the rest of the filling. Wash kale well and remove the tough center rib of each leaf. Roughly chop kale into small pieces.

4. Heat your oil, ghee, or butter in a frying pan, then add minced garlic, crushed chilies to taste, and a pinch of sea salt. Cook approximately 2 minutes until fragrant, then add your chopped kale and cook until the leaves are bright green and just starting to lose structure. Throw in your chickpeas and cook until warm. Remove from the heat.

5. Remove your squash from the oven when it is cooked through. Using a fork, scrape out the insides, which will pull away from the shell in strands, like spaghetti. Place all strands in your bowl, and toss with the kale and chickpea mixture. At this point, you can either serve it from the bowl or mix it everything together and place back in one-half of the empty squash shells for a beautiful presentation. Sprinkle with chopped toasted hazelnuts and shaved Pecorino Romano. Enjoy.

6. Serve and Enjoy!

Shakshuka (Serves 6)

<u>Ingredients:</u>

4 cups of Ripe Diced Tomatoes

1 tablespoons of Olive Oil

6 Eggs

1/2 Medium Brown or White Onion (Peeled & Diced)

1 Minced Garlic Clove

1 teaspoon of Cumin

1 Medium Green or Red Bell Pepper (Chopped)

2 tablespoons of Tomato Paste

1 teaspoon of Chili Powder (Mild)

1/2 tablespoons of Fresh Chopped Parsley

1 teaspoon of Paprika

Pinch of Cayenne Pepper

Pinch of Sugar

Salt

Pepper

Directions:

1. Heat your deep, large-sized skillet or sauté pan over a medium heat. Slowly warm olive oil in your pan. Add your chopped onion, sauté for a few minutes until the onion begins to soften. Add your garlic and continue to sauté until your mixture is fragrant.

2. Add your bell pepper, sauté for approximately 5 to 7 minutes over a medium heat until softened.

3. Add your tomatoes and tomato paste to pan, stir until blended. Add your spices and sugar, stir well, and allow mixture to simmer over a medium heat for 5 to 7 minutes until it starts to reduce. At this point, you can taste the mixture and spice it according to your preferences. Add your salt and pepper to taste, more sugar for a sweeter sauce, or more cayenne pepper for a spicier shakshuka.

4. Crack your eggs, one at a time, directly over the tomato mixture, making sure to space them evenly over the sauce. Place 5 eggs around the outer edge and 1 egg in the center. The eggs will cook "over easy" style on top of your tomato sauce.

5. Cover your pan. Allow your mixture to simmer for approximately 10 to 15 minutes, or until the eggs are cooked and the sauce has slightly reduced. Keep an eye on the skillet to make sure that the sauce doesn't reduce too much, which can lead to burning.

6. Some people prefer their shakshuka eggs runnier. If this is your preference, let the sauce reduce for a few minutes before cracking the eggs on top. Cover the pan and cook the eggs to taste.

7. Garnish with your chopped parsley, if desired.

8. Serve and Enjoy!

Chicken & Asparagus Lemon Stir Fry (Serves 4)

<u>Ingredients:</u>

1 1/2 pounds of Skinless Chicken Breast (Cut Into 1-Inch Cubes)

2 tablespoons of Reduced-Sodium Soy Sauce

1/2 cup of Reduced-Sodium Chicken Broth

2 teaspoons of Cornstarch

1 tablespoon of Canola Oil

2 tablespoons of Water

1 bunch of Asparagus (Ends Trimmed & Cut Into 2-Inch Pieces)

6 cloves of Chopped Garlic

3 tablespoons of Fresh Lemon Juice

1 tablespoon of Fresh Ginger

Fresh Black Pepper

Kosher Salt

Directions:

1. Lightly season your chicken with salt. In your small-sized bowl, combine your chicken broth and soy sauce. In a second small-sized bowl combine the cornstarch and water and mix well to combine.

2. Heat a large-sized non-stick wok over a medium-high heat, when hot add 1 teaspoon of your oil, then add the asparagus and cook until tender-crisp. Should take approximately 3 to 4 minutes. Add your garlic and ginger and cook until golden. Should take approximately 1 minute. Set to the side.

3. Increase the heat to high, then add 1 teaspoon of oil and half of the chicken and cook until browned and cooked through. Should take approximately 4 minutes on each side. Remove and set to the side and repeat with the remaining oil and chicken. Set to the side.

4. Add your soy sauce mixture; bring to a boil and cook approximately 1 1/2 minutes. Add your lemon juice and cornstarch mixture and stir well, when it simmers return the chicken and asparagus to the wok and mix well. Remove from the heat.

5. Serve and Enjoy!

Chapter Seven: Intermittent Fasting Dinner Recipes

In this section, I will share with you 10+ Intermittent Fasting dinner recipes you can prepare yourself. I'll include both beginner recipes and some advanced recipes. That way no matter what your skill level in the kitchen you'll be able to create a healthy low-calorie meal.

Chicken & Parmesan Fennel Recipe (Serves 8)

Ingredients:

3 1/2 ounces of Chicken Breast (Cut It Length-Ways)

5 ounces of Boiled Potatoes

1 teaspoon of Walnut Oil

1 tablespoon of Greek Yogurt

1/4 teaspoon of Smoked Paprika

2 teaspoons of Grated Parmesan

7 ounces of Fennel (Cut Into Eighths)

1 tablespoon of Roughly Chopped Parsley

Directions:

1. Rub your chicken with half the oil and season well with salt, pepper, and smoked paprika.

2. Preheat your oven to 390 degrees. Lay the fennel in a roasting tin with the chicken and sprinkle carefully with the Parmesan, making sure as little as possible falls in the tin. Bake for approximately 10 to 15 minutes, until browned, and the chicken is cooked through but not dried out.

3. Slice your chicken breast. Mix the last 1/2 teaspoon of walnut oil with the Greek yogurt, adding plenty of seasoning and a teaspoonful or so of water to make a thick pouring consistency.

4. Top with parsley.

5. Serve and Enjoy!

Egg Fried Rice (Serves 2)

Ingredients:

6 ounces of Basmati Rice

2 Eggs

1 tablespoon of Vegetable Oil

4 Spring Onions (Green Onions / Scallions)

4 ounces of Peas

Directions:

1. Cook your rice according to the packet instructions. Leave in your saucepan, away from the heat.

2. Heat the oil in a large-sized frying pan, and fry your eggs. Flip your eggs to fry the second side. (You're aiming for over medium consistency, and it doesn't matter if the yolks get broken.)

3. Chop your egg into small pieces.

4. Add your rice and stir into the egg.

5. Slice your spring onions, and add along with your peas.

6. Stir fry for a couple of minutes.

7. Serve and Enjoy!

Creole Cod (Serves 4)

<u>Ingredients:</u>

4 6-ounce Cod Fillets (About 1-Inch Thick)

2 teaspoons of Olive Oil

2 teaspoons of Dijon Mustard

1/2 teaspoon of Creole Seasoning Blend

1 tablespoon of Fresh Lemon Juice

1/2 teaspoon of Salt

Chopped Fresh Parsley

Cooking Spray

Directions:

1. Preheat your oven to 400 degrees.

2. Combine the first 4 ingredients. Brush evenly over fish.

3. Place your fish on a foil-lined baking sheet coated with cooking spray. Bake at 400 degrees for 17 minutes or until the fish flakes easily when tested with a fork. Drizzle juice evenly over fish. Garnish with parsley, if desired.

4. Serve it up!

Smoked Salmon & Spinach Pot (Serves 2)

Ingredients:

2 Eggs

3 1/2 ounces of Smoked Salmon

7 ounces of Spinach Leaves

1 teaspoon of Cornflour

3 1/2 ounces of Leek (Finely Chopped)

2 1/2 ounces of Low-Fat Creme Fraiche

Ground Black Pepper

Directions:

1. Cook your spinach in a tablespoon of water until wilted. Should take approximately 3 minutes. Squeeze out as much water as possible. Transfer to your bowl and add your chopped salmon, creme fraiche, leeks, cornflour, and lots of ground black pepper.

2. Put into oven proof greased ramekins. Cover each with lightly greased foil.

3. Bake at 425 degrees for approximately 15 minutes until bubbling. Take dishes out, stir well, and then make a dip in the center. Break an egg into the center of each. Cover and bake for approximately 8 minutes until your egg white is cooked but the yolk is still runny. Take dishes out, allow them to stand for 2 minutes.

4. Serve and Enjoy!

Smoked Salmon & Spinach Roulade (Serves 8)

<u>Ingredients:</u>

<u>*Spinach Cake*</u>

1 10-ounce package of Frozen Spinach (Thawed & Squeezed Dry)

2 Large Egg Yolks

6 Large Egg Whites

1/2 cup of Chopped Fresh Parsley

1/4 cup of Reduced-Fat Sour Cream

1/3 cup of Flour

Dash of Hot Pepper Sauce

Salt

Freshly Ground Pepper

<u>*Filling*</u>

6 ounces of Reduced-Fat Cream Cheese

8 ounces of Flaked Smoked Salmon

3/4 cup of Low-Fat Cottage Cheese

3 tablespoons of Drained Capers (Rinsed)

1 tablespoon of Lemon Juice

1/4 cup of Snipped Fresh Chives

Freshly Ground Pepper

Directions:

1. To make your spinach cake: Preheat your oven to 375 degrees. Coat an 11-by-17-inch rimmed baking sheet with cooking spray. Line the bottom of your baking sheet with parchment paper or wax paper and coat it with cooking spray.

2. Puree spinach, parsley, flour, sour cream and hot pepper sauce in your food processor until smooth. Season with salt and pepper. Add your egg yolks and pulse to mix. Transfer to your bowl and set to the side.

3. Beat egg whites in your mixing bowl with an electric mixer until stiff, but not dry, peaks form. Fold 1/3 of the beaten whites into your spinach puree with a rubber spatula to lighten it. Fold your spinach mixture into the remaining whites until blended and spread in your prepared pan. Bake until the top springs back when lightly touched. Should take approximately 8 to 10 minutes. Allow it to cool in the pan on a rack for approximately 5 minutes.

4. Cover the work surface with a clean kitchen towel with the long edge toward you. Invert your spinach cake onto the towel. Peel off the parchment or wax paper and cover your spinach cake with another towel.

5. Puree cream cheese and cottage cheese in a food processor until smooth. Transfer to your small-sized bowl and set to the side.

6. Uncover your spinach cake and sprinkle the surface with lemon juice. Leaving a little border to accommodate the filling, spread half of the cheese mixture on the spinach cake and distribute smoked salmon evenly on top. Spread the remaining cheese mixture over the salmon. Sprinkle with chives and capers. Season with pepper.

7. Starting at the long edge, gently roll your cake and filling as you would roll a jelly roll, using the towel to lift and assist in the rolling. Wrap the roulade in plastic wrap and refrigerate for at least 4 hours.

8. Cut your roulade into 24 slices with a serrated knife.

9. Serve and Enjoy!

Mixed Vegetable Frittata (Serves 4)

Ingredients:

7 Medium Eggs

3 1/2 ounces of Cheddar Cheese

1 ounce of Parmesan Cheese

3 Small Red Onions

1 Sweet Red Pepper

4 Large Chestnut Mushrooms

1 Medium Courgette

8 spears of Asparagus

1 teaspoon of Olive Oil

Black Pepper

Directions:

1. Chop all of your vegetables (fairly thin slices/small pieces), and grate the cheeses.

2. Heat the oil in your large-sized frying pan and fry your vegetables over a medium heat until tender.

3. Meanwhile, break your eggs into a bowl and mix them with a fork. Add pepper to the eggs and stir.

4. Pour your eggs into the pan with the vegetables and turn the mixture a few times to combine. (The egg will start to cook as you're doing this.)

5. Leave to cook over a low heat until the top of the frittata is set. Should take approximately 10 minutes.

6. Sprinkle the cheeses evenly over the top of your frittata and put under a hot grill for a couple of minutes to melt the cheese and cook the top.

7. Serve and Enjoy!

Cajun Chicken Kebab (Serves 2)

Ingredients:

2 Chicken Breasts (Skinless & Cut Into Chunks)

2 Weight Watchers Pitta Bread

3 1/2 ounces of Low Fat Natural Yogurt

1 Medium Tomato (Thinly Sliced)

1 teaspoon of Cajun Spice

1 Small Red Onion (Peeled & Thinly Sliced)

1 1/2 ounces of Fresh Rocket Leaves

1/4 teaspoon of Ground Coriander

1/4 teaspoon of Ground Cumin

1 Lemon (Cut In Half & One Half Cut Into 2 Wedges)

Pepper

Salt

Directions:

1. Spoon about a quarter of your low-fat yogurt into a bowl and add your Cajun spice mix, and the juice of half a lemon. Mix together well and then add the chicken pieces and allow to marinate for at least an hour or up to four hours.

2. Just before cooking, take the chicken pieces out of the marinade. Heat a griddle pan over a medium heat and put the chicken pieces in the pan. Keep moving them around so they don't stick to the pan and keep cooking over a low heat until cooked.

3. Mix the rest of the low-fat yogurt with the ground coriander and cumin, and spoon into a small-sized bowl.

4. Two or three minutes before the chicken is cooked, pop the pitta bread in a toaster or in a warm oven and heat them up. Arrange your rocket leaves, sliced tomatoes and sliced red onion on a plate.

5. Divide your chicken pieces between two plates and allow your diners to assemble the kebab themselves by adding your salad and yogurt dip to the chicken in a split pitta bread.

6. Serve and Enjoy!

Black Bean & Corn Fajitas (Serves 2)

Ingredients:

10 ounces of Black Beans (Cooked & Drained)

2 tablespoons of Olive Oil

1 Zucchini

1 Large Onion

1 Red Bell Pepper

6 ounces of Sweetcorn

4 tablespoons of Fajita Spice Mix

8 Tortilla Wraps

Thick Sour Cream

Salsa

Directions:

1. Slice the zucchini, red pepper, and onion into thin strips.

2. Heat the oil in your large-sized frying pan and add the vegetables and spices.

3. Stir fry until your vegetables are soft and coated in the spice mixture. Add your black beans and corn and cook over a medium heat until warmed through.

4. Gently warm your tortillas.

5. Add sour cream, salsa, and a crunchy salad on the side.

6. Serve and Enjoy!

Creamy Mushroom Farfalle (Serves 4)

<u>Ingredients:</u>

2 Large Onions

2 1/2 cups of Chestnut Mushrooms

1 Small Leek

2 tablespoons of Ground Almonds

6 cloves of Garlic

1 1/2 cups of Wholemeal Farfalle

1 cup of Double Cream

1/2 teaspoon of Cinnamon

1/2 teaspoon of Nutmeg

4 tablespoons of Fresh Parsley

Black Pepper

Butter

<u>Directions:</u>

1. Finely chop your onion, leek, and garlic. Saute in a butter, until soft.

2. Chop your mushrooms and add to the pan with your onions. Continue to saute over a low heat until your mushrooms are cooked.

3. Add your cream, ground almonds, parsley, and spices. Season generously with black pepper.

4. Simmer your sauce over a low heat, and meanwhile, cook your pasta according to the instructions on the packet.

5. Serve with extra parsley to garnish.

6. Serve and Enjoy!

Spicy Vegetable Stir-Fry (Serves 2)

Ingredients:

Zucchini Ribbons:

2 Large Zucchini

2 teaspoons of Sesame Seeds

2 teaspoons of Sesame Oil

Stir-Fry:

1 Large Red Onion

3 1/2 ounces of Sugar Snap Peas

4 1/2 ounces of Baby Corn

1/2 teaspoon of Ground Ginger

2 Red Pointed Peppers

5 1/4 ounces of Chestnut Mushrooms

5 1/4 ounces of Beans Sprouts

2 tablespoons of Soy Sauce

1 teaspoon of Chili Flakes

2 cloves of Garlic

<u>Directions:</u>

1. Make zucchini ribbons by running your potato peeler from top to bottom of the zucchini (stop when you reach the seeds in the middle). Set to the side.

2. Cut your mushrooms into thick slices and your peppers into strips. Cut your baby corn in half. Finely chop the red onion and garlic.

3. Stir-fry your vegetables (except for the onions and garlic) for approximately 5 minutes, until soft.

4. Add your onions, spices, garlic, and soy sauce. Cook for approximately 2 to 3 minutes.

5. Meanwhile, cook your zucchini ribbons by microwaving in a bowl for approximately 2 to 3 minutes. Drain your liquid from the zucchini and toss in the sesame oil and sesame seeds.

6. Serve and Enjoy!

Salmon, Cream Cheese, & Dill Souffle (Serves 8)

Ingredients:

4 Large Egg Yolks (At Room Temperature)

8 Large Egg Whites (At Room Temperature)

4 ounces of Smoked Salmon (Chopped)

3 tablespoons of Fine Dry Breadcrumbs

2 tablespoons of Unsalted Butter

1 1/2 cups of Low-Fat Milk

2 tablespoons of Canola Oil

2 tablespoons of Chopped Fresh or Dried Dill

1/4 cup of All-Purpose Flour

4 ounces of Reduced-Fat Cream Cheese (Softened)

1/4 teaspoon of Freshly Ground Pepper

1/8 teaspoon of Salt

Directions:

1. Position rack in lower third of your oven. Preheat your oven to 375 degrees. Coat eight 10-ounce ramekins or a 2 1/2-quart souffle with cooking spray. Sprinkle with enough breadcrumbs to generously coat the inside, tilting to evenly distribute. Tap out any excess. Place ramekins on your baking sheet.

2. Heat your milk in a small-sized saucepan over a medium heat until steaming. Melt your butter and oil in a medium-sized saucepan over a medium-low heat. Whisk in your flour and cook, whisking, for 2 minutes. Slowly whisk in your hot milk and cook over a medium-low heat whisking, until the mixture is the consistency of thick batter. Should take approximately 2 to 4 minutes. Transfer to your large-sized bowl. Whisk in egg yolks, one at a time, until incorporated. Whisk in your cream cheese until melted, then stir in your salmon, dill, and pepper.

3. Clean and dry a large-sized mixing bowl and beaters, making sure there are no traces of oil. (Any fat in your egg whites may prevent your souffle from rising properly.) Beat your egg whites in the bowl with an electric mixer on medium speed until foamy. Add your salt. Gradually increase speed to high and beat until shiny and stiff, but not dry. Do not over beat. Stop when your egg whites hold their shape in the bowl and on the beater but don't look overly dry or lumpy.

4. Using your rubber spatula, stir one-third of the whites into your egg-yolk mixture to lighten it. Gently fold in your remaining egg whites until evenly distributed. It's normal if a few white streaks remain. Spoon your batter into the prepared dish(es).

5. Bake until puffed and firm to the touch. Should take approximately 20 to 24 minutes for 10-ounce souffles and approximately 38 to 42 minutes for a 2 1/2-quart souffle. (Resist the temptation to take a peek until the last 5 minutes of baking. An open oven door will let in too much cool air and may interrupt the rising.)

6. Once out of your oven, even a beautifully puffed souffle will slowly deflate, so go directly to the table.

7. Serve and Enjoy!

Fast Ciabatta Pizza (Serves 4)

Ingredients:

3 1/2 ounces of Grated Mozzarella Cheese

3/4 cup of Tomato Sauce

1 packet of Ciabatta Bread Mix

8 Chestnut Mushrooms

1/2 Zucchini

1 Red Pepper

1/2 cup of Sweetcorn

Directions:

1. Make up your Ciabatta mix according to the packet instructions. Roll out the dough to about 1 centimeter thick, on a large floured baking sheet. Leave to rest for half an hour.

2. While your dough is resting, slice your vegetables and grate your cheese.

3. Knock back the dough, prick the surface with your fork, and spread your tomato sauce evenly.

4. Arrange your vegetables on top of the sauce. Sprinkle cheese over your vegetables.

5. Cook for approximately 15 minutes in a 425-degree oven.

6. Serve and Enjoy!

Veggie Pasta Bake (Serves 4)

Ingredients:

1 1/4 cups of Pasta

2 tablespoons of Olive Oil

1 Large Onion

1 Red Pepper

1 Courgette

1 cup of Grated Mature Cheddar Cheese

4 1/2 ounces of Sweetcorn

2 1/2 ounces of Cream Cheese

4 Cherry Tomatoes

Mushrooms

Basil

Oregano

Directions:

1. Preheat the oven to 400 degrees.

2. Heat your olive oil in a large-sized casserole dish in your oven.

3. Finely chop your vegetables, add to your hot oil (except for the sweetcorn), and return to the oven for approximately 15 minutes.

4. Meanwhile, cook your pasta according to the instructions on the packet.

5. Toss your pasta, vegetables, sweetcorn, and herbs in the casserole dish with the cream cheese and half the cheddar.

6. Sprinkle the remaining cheese on top, and arrange your cherry tomatoes (halved) on the top.

7. Bake for approximately 15 minutes, or until your cheese has started to bubble and brown.

8. Serve and Enjoy!

Creamy Paprika Rigatoni (Serves 2)

Ingredients:

8 ounces of Rigatoni Pasta

1 Large Onion

6 ounces of Chestnut Button Mushrooms

1 Red Bell Pepper

3 tablespoons of Boiling Water

1 teaspoon of Olive Oil

1 Low-Sodium Stock Cube

3 tablespoons of Plain Greek Yogurt

1 tablespoon of Tomato Puree (Concentrated)

1/2 teaspoon of Smoked Paprika

Directions:

1. Chop your onion and pepper into bite-sized pieces. Cut the button mushrooms in half.

2. Cook your pasta according to your packet instructions.

3. Meanwhile, heat your olive oil in a medium-sized saucepan, and saute the vegetables until soft.

4. Dissolve your stock cube in the boiling water, and add to the vegetables along with the tomato puree, yogurt, and paprika.

5. Simmer your sauce over a low heat until it is warmed through.

6. Drain your pasta and quickly toss through your sauce.

7. Serve and Enjoy!

Carrot & Broccoli Pasta (Serves 4)

Ingredients:

1 3/4 cups of Pasta

4 Large Carrots

1 Small Head of Broccoli

2 tablespoons of Olive Oil

1 tin of Red Kidney Beans

3 tablespoons of Lemon Juice

Salt

Black Pepper

Directions:

1. Prepare your vegetables: chop your carrots into circular slices and your broccoli into florets.

2. Bring a large-sized pan of water to the boil.

3. The carrots will need 10 minutes in total (assuming you like them al dente), so look at your pasta packet and subtract your pasta cooking time from this to work out when to add the pasta. (For very heavy pasta you might need to add the pasta first, but normally it will be at the same time or a little after.)

4. With 5 minutes remaining, add your broccoli florets to the pan.

5. Add the red kidney beans (well rinsed) with a couple of minutes to spare.

6. Toss through your olive oil, and season with lemon juice, salt, and pepper.

7. Serve and Enjoy!

Spinach Fettuccine Alfredo (Serves 2)

<u>Ingredients:</u>

1/4 cup of Pine Nuts

6 ounces of Fettuccine

3 tablespoons of Pecorino Cheese

1 tablespoon of Butter

2/3 cup of Double Cream

1 Large Shallot

1 Egg Yolk

2 teaspoons of Lemon Juice

4 ounces of Fresh Spinach

2 teaspoons of Ground Black Pepper

<u>Directions:</u>

1. Cook your pasta according to packet instructions.

2. While your pasta is cooking, make the Alfredo sauce.

3. Finely chop your shallot.

4. Melt your butter in a small-sized frying pan and fry the shallot until softened.

5. In a separate dry saucepan, toast your pine nuts over a medium heat, turning occasionally.

6. Whisk together your cream and egg yolk.

7. Add your cream mixture to the pan with the shallot and cook for approximately 2 to 3 minutes until your sauce begins to thicken.

8. Season with your grated cheese, pepper, and lemon juice.

9. Drain your pasta, reserving a little of the cooking water.

10. Stir your spinach into the sauce to wilt, and then stir into the pasta. Use a little of the reserved water to loosen the texture if necessary.

11. Sprinkle with toasted pine nuts.

12. Serve and Enjoy!

Chapter Eight: Intermittent Fasting Soups, Sides, & Snacks Recipes

In this section, I will share with you 10+ Intermittent Fasting side dish recipes you can prepare yourself. I'll include both beginner recipes and some advanced recipes. That way no matter what your skill level in the kitchen you'll be able to create a healthy low-calorie side dish.

Mushroom Miso Soup (Serves 1)

Ingredients:

2 cups of Mushroom Stock

4 Small Chestnut Mushrooms

1 tablespoon of Miso Paste

2 Spring Onions (Scallions /Green Onions)

3 1/2 ounces of Tofu

Directions:

1. Heat your mushroom stock and dissolve in your miso paste.

2. Chop your tofu and mushrooms into small bite-sized pieces and slice the spring onions.

3. Add the tofu and vegetables to the broth and simmer for approximately five minutes until heated through.

4. Serve and Enjoy!

Twice Baked Potatoes

Ingredients:

4 Large Baked Potatoes

3 1/2 ounces of Grated Cheddar Cheese

1 Large Red Onion

1 Leek

1 tablespoon of Olive Oil

Directions:

1. Preheat your oven to 400 degrees.

2. Meanwhile, slice your leek and onion finely. Fry them in a little olive oil.

3. Once your leek and onion have softened, slice your potatoes in half and carefully scrape the potato out of the skins.

4. Add your potato to a large-sized mixing bowl with the leek, onion, and grated cheese. Mash until well combined.

5. Stuff your potato skins with the mixture, pressing down firmly as it will be a tight fit.

6. Place on your baking tray in the oven and bake for approximately 10 to 15 minutes, until the top is beginning to crisp.

7. Serve and Enjoy!

Butternut Squash & Spinach Risotto (Serves 2)

Ingredients:

10 ounces of Butternut Squash

7 ounces of Arborio Risotto Rice

1 Large Red Onion

2 cloves of Garlic

3 1/2 ounces of Spinach

1 Red Sweet Pepper

1 teaspoon of Olive Oil

1 pint of Vegetable Stock

Handful of Flat Leaf Parsley

Black Pepper

Directions:

1. Peel your squash, scrape out the seeds and cut into cubes around 1/2-inch across.

2. Finely chop your onion, garlic, and red pepper.

3. Wash and roughly chop your spinach.

4. Heat your oil in a large-sized heavy saucepan.

5. Fry your squash, onion, garlic, and red pepper together over a low/medium heat until the squash starts to soften.

6. Add your rice and stock. Simmer for approximately 15 to 20 minutes, stirring frequently and adding additional hot water as required to keep the rice from boiling dry.

7. Season liberally with your black pepper.

8. Once your rice is cooked, add your spinach and fresh parsley. Stir it through until the leaves wilt.

9. Serve and Enjoy!

Summer Vegetable Soup (Serves 4)

Ingredients:

2 Large Onions

1 tablespoon of Olive Oil

1 Leek

2 liters of Vegetable Stock

1 Zucchini

1 Red Pepper

1 cup of Peas

4 Carrots

1/2 Broccoli

1/2 Cauliflower

1/2 Savoy Cabbage

Directions:

1. Chop all your vegetables.

2. Heat the oil in a large-sized saucepan and fry your leek, onions, pepper, and zucchini until soft.

3. Add your stock and carrots. Simmer for approximately 15 minutes.

4. Add your remaining vegetables and simmer until your broccoli is soft.

5. Serve and Enjoy!

Butternut Squash & Split Pea Soup (Serves 2)

<u>Ingredients:</u>

11 ounces of Butternut Squash Flesh

4 teaspoons of Hungarian Paprika

1 teaspoon of Olive Oil

1 Onion

8 ounces of Yellow Split Peas (Dry Weight)

4 cloves of Garlic

1 3/4 pints of Vegetable Stock

Black Pepper

<u>Directions:</u>

1. Peel and chop your butternut squash.

2. Heat your oil in a large, deep saucepan.

3. Fry your onion, garlic, and squash until your onion is soft.

4. Add the split peas and stock. Season with paprika and black pepper.

5. Simmer for about an hour, until the split peas are cooked (it can take as long as two hours; to speed it up, soak your peas overnight).

6. Use a potato masher to puree your squash.

7. Sprinkle with some paprika.

8. Serve and Enjoy!

Thai Mushroom Soup (Serves 4)

Ingredients:

9 ounces of Field Mushrooms

7 ounces of Chestnut Mushrooms

3 1/2 ounces of Baby Button Mushrooms

2 Large Onions

1 teaspoon of Toasted Sesame Oil

6 Large Garlic Cloves

1 tablespoon of Tomato Puree

1 Small Red Chili

1 3/4 ounces of Coconut Cream

2 tablespoons of Red Thai Curry Paste

3/4 ounce of Fresh Chopped Cilantro

2 pints of Boiling Water

Fresh Ginger (1-Inch)

Directions:

1. Finely chop your onions and field mushrooms. Fry in the sesame oil for approximately 10 minutes until soft.

2. Chop your ginger, garlic, and chili. Stir into the onion/mushroom mixture and fry for a couple more minutes.

3. Add your curry paste, tomato puree, and around 1/2 pint of boiling water. Simmer over a low heat for approximately 45 minutes.

4. Dissolve your coconut cream into the soup and add the rest of the boiling water.

5. Trim the button mushrooms and cut the chestnut mushrooms into thick slices. Add these to the soup, along with the chopped cilantro. Simmer for a further 5 minutes until all your mushrooms are tender.

6. Stir the cilantro through just before serving, and reserve a little to garnish.

7. Serve and Enjoy!

Red & White Quinoa Bowl (Serves 2)

Ingredients:

7 ounces of Mushrooms

2 ounces of White Quinoa

1 1/2 ounces of Red Quinoa

1 tablespoon of Wholegrain Mustard

2 Red Pointed Peppers

1 tablespoon of Lemon Juice

Directions:

1. Cook your quinoa according to the instructions on the packet.

2. Chop your peppers into large-sized chunks and quarter your mushrooms.

3. Mix your lemon juice and mustard together.

4. Add your vegetables and the lemon/mustard to a frying pan. Saute over a medium heat for approximately 5 minutes until softened.

5. Add your quinoa to the pan with the vegetables and toss through to coat in the lemon dressing.

6. Serve and Enjoy!

Italian Stuffed Mushrooms (Serves 2)

<u>Ingredients:</u>

6 Large Chestnut Mushrooms

1 ounce of Grated Cheddar Cheese

2 cloves of Garlic

1 ounce of Fine Breadcrumbs

1 Small Onion

2 tablespoons of White Wine

1 tablespoon of Olive Oil

Handful of Fresh Herbs (Oregano & Thyme)

<u>Directions:</u>

1. Preheat your oven to 390 degrees.

2. Remove the stalks from your mushrooms.

3. Wash your mushroom caps, pat dry with a sheet of kitchen paper and arrange in a non-stick roasting tray.

4. Finely chop the garlic, onion, and mushroom stalks.

5. Heat the oil in your small-sized pan and sauté the garlic, onion, and mushroom stalks until soft.

6. Add your wine and simmer for a couple of minutes.

7. Stir in your breadcrumbs.

8. Spoon your mixture into the mushroom caps.

9. Bake for approximately 10 to 15 minutes, until the mushrooms are cooked through.

10. Serve and Enjoy!

 # Turkish-Inspired Casserole Recipe (Serves 6)

Ingredients:

1 Large Zucchini

1 Medium Aubergine

3 Medium Tomatoes

1 Leek

1 Red Pepper

1 Green Pepper

1 Medium Onion

6 Small Mushrooms

1 tablespoon of Oregano

2 tablespoons of Tomato Puree

1 teaspoon of Sumac

1 tablespoon of Parsley

2 handfuls of Spinach

Directions:

1. Chop your zucchini, aubergine, and peppers into small pieces (about 1/2-inch square). Slice your leeks and onion. Cut mushrooms in half. Cut tomatoes into eighths.

2. Fry the aubergine for 5 minutes over a medium heat.

3. Add your courgette, peppers, onion, and leeks. Fry until softened.

4. Add tomato puree, tomatoes, mushrooms, and seasonings.

5. Add to a lidded casserole dish, and bake for approximately 15 minutes at 400 degrees.

6. Stir in your spinach and bake for an additional 15 minutes.

7. Serve and Enjoy!

Vegetarian Puttanesca Sauce (Serves 2)

Ingredients:

20 Large Kalamata Olives

3 tablespoons of Olive Oil

1 Large Onion

1 tablespoon of Capers

2 cloves of Garlic

1 1/2 cups of Tomato Sauce

Directions:

1. Chop your onion and crush your garlic.

2. Heat your oil in a large-sized frying pan and fry your onion and garlic until soft.

3. Add your tomato sauce, olives, and capers. Simmer for approximately 15 to 20 minutes to infuse the flavors.

4. Add over pasta.

5. Serve and Enjoy!

Mexican Quinoa Stuffed Peppers (Serves 3)

Ingredients:

6 Bell Peppers

1 Small Red Onion

2 teaspoons of Olive Oil

5 ounces of Sweetcorn

5 ounces of Cherry Tomatoes

9 ounces of Cooked Quinoa (1 packet)

1 tablespoon of Diced Jalapeños

2 tablespoons of Fresh Coriander

Juice of 1 Lime

1 3/4 ounces of Grated Cheese (Optional)

Directions:

1. Preheat your oven to 400 degrees.

2. Wash your peppers, cut the tops off with a sharp knife and scoop out the seeds.

3. Rub the outside of your peppers with olive oil and arrange on your baking tray.

4. Finely dice your red onion and quarter the cherry tomatoes.

5. Mix your onion, tomatoes, quinoa, sweetcorn, lime juice, coriander, jalapeños, and cheese (if using) in a large-sized bowl.

6. Fill the peppers with your quinoa mixture and replace the pepper tops.

7. Bake for approximately 25 to 30 minutes, until the pepper skins are starting to blacken.

8. Serve and Enjoy!

Spiced Cauliflower (Serves 2)

<u>Ingredients:</u>

21 ounces of Cauliflower

5 1/4 ounces of Chestnut Mushrooms

1/2 Red Pepper

7 ounces of Vegetable Stock

1 Small Onion

3 1/2 ounces of Cherry Tomatoes

1 teaspoon of Sunflower Oil

4 cloves of Garlic

1/2 teaspoon of Turmeric

2 teaspoons of Garam Masala

4 Cardamom Pods

Directions:

1. Cut the cauliflower into florets. Roughly chop your onion, pepper, and mushrooms. Cut your tomatoes in half. Finely dice the garlic.

2. Heat your oil in a large-sized saucepan.

3. Fry your onion, pepper, and garlic until the onions are soft.

4. Add your spices and mushrooms and fry for a couple more minutes.

5. Add your vegetable stock and cauliflower florets. Simmer for about 10 minutes over a medium heat, turning regularly to coat all the cauliflower florets in the spiced stock.

6. Add your tomatoes, cover, and simmer gently for another couple of minutes to soften the tomatoes.

7. Serve up with a slotted spoon to leave behind any excess liquid.

8. Serve and Enjoy!

Date & Brazil Energy Bars (Serves 20)

Ingredients:

2 cups of Whole Dates

1 cup of Brazil Nuts

1 cup of Raisins

1 cup of Apricots

2 tablespoons of Sesame Seeds

2 tablespoons of Golden Linseeds

Directions:

1. Finely chop your Brazil nuts in your food processor. Remove to a large-sized mixing bowl.

2. Whiz your dates, apricots, and raisins in your food processor until fairly smooth (a few smaller lumps are fine).

3. Add your pureed fruit to the mixing bowl, along with the nuts and add your seeds.

4. Knead your mixture until your nuts and seeds are evenly distributed.

5. Line a tray bake tin with your greaseproof paper and push the fruit mixture into the pan from one end, compressing it as much as you can by hand.

6. Chill in your refrigerator for an hour.

7. Top with more greaseproof paper, find something large and flat (like a chopping board) that fits within your tray bake tin and use to compress the mixture by piling with heavy objects such as books.

8. After a few hours, you should be able to neatly cut the bars with a sharp knife.

9. Serve and Enjoy!

Chapter Nine: Intermittent Fasting Dessert Recipes

In this section, I will share with you 10+ Intermittent Fasting dessert recipes you can prepare yourself. I'll include both beginner recipes and some advanced recipes. That way no matter what your skill level in the kitchen you'll be able to create a healthy low-calorie meal.

Simple Cheesecake (Serves 10)

<u>Ingredients:</u>

2 1/2 ounces of Ginger Biscuits

7 ounces of Cream Cheese

2 ounces of Digestive Biscuits

3/5 cup of Double Cream

1 3/4 ounces of Butter

1 3/4 ounces of Icing Sugar

Half a Vanilla Pod

Fruit of Choice

<u>Directions:</u>

1. Line the base of a 6-inch loose-bottomed baking tin with a circle of greaseproof paper.

2. Put your biscuits in a large-sized mixing bowl and crush with the end of a rolling pin.

3. Melt your butter and stir in the crumbs until thoroughly combined. Press your mixture into the base of the tin and refrigerate for approximately 1 hour.

4. In a clean bowl, whip the cream until stiff.

5. Split the vanilla pod with a sharp knife and scrape out the seeds.

6. Combine your cream cheese, icing sugar, and vanilla seeds (you can use the same bowl as you used for the biscuits if you wipe out any spare crumbs).

7. Fold in the whipped cream and whisk your mixture for a few more minutes.

8. Spoon your cheese mixture onto the biscuit base, and smooth the top with your spatula.

9. Refrigerate for a few hours. Take out of refrigerator and top with your choice of fresh or canned fruit.

10. Serve and Enjoy!

Cherry Chocolate Cookies (Serves 24)

Ingredients:

3 cups of Flour

9 ounces of Butter

1/2 cup of Cacao Powder

2 Eggs

1 cup of Molasses Sugar

2/3 cup of Soft Brown Sugar

1 teaspoon of Vanilla Essence

1 teaspoon of Baking Powder

1 1/2 cups of Glace Cherries (Halved)

Directions:

1. Preheat your oven to 320 degrees.

2. Combine your dry ingredients in your large-sized mixing bowl.

3. Melt your butter and add to your bowl along with the eggs and vanilla essence.

4. Knead together into a soft dough.

5. Add the cherries and knead until evenly distributed.

6. Use a dessert spoon to scoop out cookie mixture, form into a ball between your fingers and arrange on baking sheets.

7. Bake for approximately 15 to 20 minutes until starting to firm.

8. Cool on a wire rack before serving.

9. Serve and Enjoy!

Chocolate Box Cake (Serves 16)

Ingredients:

Cake:

8 ounces of Plain Flour

1 1/2 tablespoons of Baking Powder

4 ounces of Caster Sugar

4 ounces of Cocoa Powder

1/2 pint of Hot Water

2 tablespoons of Instant Coffee Granules

7 tablespoons of Sunflower Oil

1 tablespoon of Molasses

1 tablespoon of Vanilla Bean Extract

Butter Cream:

4 ounces of Butter

8 ounce of Icing Sugar

1 ounce of Cocoa powder

2 tablespoons of Water

1 teaspoon of Vanilla Bean Extract

Decoration:

12 ounces of Golden Marzipan

16 Chocolates

Directions:

1. Preheat your oven to 350 degrees and line a 7-inch square cake tin.

2. Sieve together the flour, cocoa powder, caster sugar, and baking powder for your cake.

3. Dissolve the coffee granules and molasses in the hot water.

4. Add to the flour, along with the oil and vanilla and stir until no dry patches remain.

5. Pour your cake mix into the tin and bake for approximately 30 to 40 minutes, or until a knife comes out clean.

6. Remove your cake from the tin and set aside to cool on a wire rack.

7. Once the cake is completely cold, you're ready to decorate it.

8. Slice the cake in half with a sharp knife and optionally also slice a little off the top to flatten the surface.

9. Make the butter cream by first softening the butter to room temperature and beating with an electric whisk.

10. Gradually fold in the icing sugar, cocoa powder, and vanilla.

11. Once the icing is folded in, beat the mixture until light and fluffy.

12. Spread half of the butter cream onto the bottom half of the cake, smooth it out, and sandwich the top half of the cake back into position.

13. Spread the remaining butter cream across the top of the cake, mounding a little in the corners if necessary to create a flatter surface.

14. Roll about half of the marzipan into a square just slightly larger than your cake and place on top of the cake.

15. Arrange the chocolates in a grid formation.

16. Roll 4 thick sausages of marzipan to make the outer edges of the box. Roll 8 thin sausages to create the internal dividers.

17. Next, check the height and width measurements of your cake, and cut cardboard pieces to the appropriate size. Tape the cardboard together into a frame which should just lift on and off the cake (to allow for cutting).

18. Decorate with a wide ribbon tied into a bow.

19. Serve and Enjoy!

Raisin & Apple Cookies (Serves 12)

Ingredients:

1 1/2 cup of Plain Flour

1 Egg

3/4 cup of Soft Brown Sugar

1 stick of Butter

1/2 teaspoon of Baking Powder

1/2 teaspoon of Vanilla Essence

1 teaspoon of Cinnamon

1/2 cup of Raisins

1/2 cup of Apple Pieces (1 Medium Cooking Apple Chopped Finely)

Directions:

1. Preheat your oven to 320 degrees.

2. Mix your dry ingredients breaking up any lumps.

3. Melt your butter.

4. Break the egg into your butter, along with the vanilla essence and mix with a fork until even.

5. Add your liquids, apple, and raisins to your dry ingredients.

6. Knead until you reach a dough of even consistency.

7. Divide into balls and press lightly onto a baking tray. Allow space for the cookies to spread during baking.

8. Bake for approximately 15 to 20 minutes until golden brown.

9. Cool on a wire rack.

10. Serve and Enjoy!

Lemon Drizzle Cake

<u>Ingredients:</u>

<u>Cake:</u>

6 ounces Sugar

2 Eggs

4 ounces of Butter

6 ounces of Self-Raising Flour

Zest of 1 Lemon

<u>Topping:</u>

2 ounces of Icing Sugar

2 teaspoons of Granulated Sugar

Juice of 1 Lemon

Directions:

1. Preheat the oven to 330 degrees. Grease your medium-sized loaf tin.

2. Cream your butter and sugar together with a spoon. Break 2 eggs into your bowl and stir until the mixture is smooth.

3. Fold in your flour and lemon zest.

4. Spoon your cake mixture into the tin, smooth with a spatula, and bake for approximately 50 minutes.

5. When your cake is about 10 minutes away from done, it's time to make the topping. Combine your icing sugar and lemon juice in a small-sized saucepan and simmer gently to reduce.

6. Take the cake out of the oven. The crust should be golden-brown and a skewer should come out clean. Remove from your tin onto a cooling tray.

7. Prick the top of the cake in several places, then gently spoon your lemon mixture over the top of the cake (before it has a chance to cool down). Sprinkle a little extra granulated sugar on top for added crunch.

8. Serve and Enjoy!

Chocolate & Rose Cupcakes (Serves 4)

Ingredients:

Cakes:

4 ounces of Butter

2 Eggs

4 ounces of Caster Sugar

4 ounces of Self-Raising Flour

3 1/1 ounces of Dark Chocolate Chips

1 teaspoon of Rose Water

Icing:

6 tablespoons of Icing Sugar

1 tablespoon of Boiling Water

Red or Pink Food Coloring

Directions:

1. Line 10 holes of a small muffin tin with paper or silicone cake liners and preheat the oven to 340 degrees.

2. Cream your butter and sugar together with the back of your spoon.

3, Add your eggs one by one, whisking until combined, then stir in your rose essence.

4. Beat your mixture until light and bubbly.

5. Gently fold in your flour, until fully combined, then add your chocolate chips.

6. Divide your cake mix between the cake cases.

7. Bake for approximately 15 to 20 minutes, or until the surface is springy and a knife comes out clean. Remove from the tin to cool on a wire rack.

8. Once the cakes have cooled to room temperature, make your icing. Dissolve your icing sugar in the boiling water and add a drop of food coloring.

9. Spoon a little icing on top of each cake, spread out with the back of your teaspoon. Allow them to set.

10. Serve and Enjoy!

Coconut Ice (Serves 64)

Ingredients:

14 ounces of Condensed Milk

14 ounces of Desiccated Coconut

10 1/2 ounces of Icing Sugar

Red Food Coloring

Directions:

1. Empty your condensed milk into your large-sized mixing bowl and add your icing sugar. Stir until your mixture is smooth.

2. Add your coconut and mix together well. You may want to knead it with your hands.

3. Line your 8-inch square dish with greaseproof paper.

4. Divide your coconut mixture in half and press half of it into the bottom of your tin, smoothing it with your hands or a spatula to give a level surface.

5. Use a small amount of food coloring to color the remainder of your mixture pink.

6. Press your remaining coconut mixture into your tin to create a second layer. Again, level the surface.

7. Refrigerate for a couple of hours. Cut into 1-inch squares and spread out to allow them to dry out further.

8. Serve and Enjoy!

Mini Florentine Bites (Serves 30)

Ingredients:

3 1/2 ounces of Dark Chocolate

15 Hazelnuts

8 Cherries

8 Pecan Nuts

Candied Peel

Toasted Flaked Almonds

Directions:

1. Start melting your chocolate.

2. Meanwhile, chop your hazelnuts in half and cut your pecans and cherries into quarters.

3. Divide your melted chocolate between 30 silicone cake cases, or (if you don't have these) make drops onto a large-sized sheet of greaseproof paper.

4. Before the chocolate hardens, arrange on each chocolate disc: 1/2 hazelnut, 1/4 pecan nut, 1/4 cherry, a couple of pieces of candied peel, and an almond flake.

5. Allow it to cool and chill in the fridge before serving.

6. Serve and Enjoy!

Apple Lattice Pie (Serves 8)

Ingredients:

Pastry:

9 ounces of Flour

1 ounce of Caster Sugar

1 Egg Yolk

4 1/2 ounces of Butter

Cold Water

Filling:

5 Large Apples

2 teaspoons of Cinnamon

3 1/2 ounces of Sultanas

1 3/4 ounces of Caster Sugar

Finish:

Milk

1 tablespoon of Golden Granulated Sugar

Directions:

1. Preheat your oven to 400 degrees and grease a 9-inch pie dish.

2. Make your pastry: Mix the flour and caster sugar together. Cut in the butter to form crumbs. Add your egg yolk, a little cold water and pull together to form a dough. Keep adding cold water, a little at a time, until the pastry sticks together.

3. Peel and chop your apples. The chunks don't have to be all the same size.

4. In your large-sized saucepan, heat the apples over a medium heat with your cinnamon, sugar, and sultanas. (No need to add any fat or liquid.) Cook until your apples have softened. Set aside to cool.

5. Roll 2/3 of the pastry into a circle to line the pie dish.

6. Fill the pie dish with your apple mixture.

7. Roll your remaining pastry into a rectangle and cut strips approximately 1/2-inch thick. You'll need strips of different lengths - I used four about the diameter of the pie dish and four shorter ones. Longer strips can always be trimmed after you've interleaved them.

8. Weave a lattice on top of the pie and fasten down the edges with a little water (after finishing the lattice pattern).

9. Brush the top of your pastry with a little milk or water. Sprinkle your granulated sugar over the top and bake for approximately 40 to 50 minutes.

10. Serve and Enjoy!

White Chocolate Berry Cheesecake (Serves 8)

Ingredients:

5 1/4 ounces of Digestive Biscuits

2 1/4 ounces of Butter

10 1/2 ounces of Raspberries

5 1/4 ounces of Strawberries

5 1/4 ounces of White Chocolate

14 ounces of Cream Cheese

6 3/4 fl. ounces of Double Cream

1 teaspoon of Pure Vanilla Extract

2 ounces of Icing Sugar

Directions:

1. Use greaseproof paper to line the base of a 7-inch loose-bottomed cake tin.

2. Crush your biscuits, melt the butter and stir in the crumbs until thoroughly combined. Press your mixture into the base of the cake tin and refrigerate for an hour.

3. Reserve enough fruit to fully cover the top of your cheesecake and chop the remainder onto the chilled biscuit base.

4. Melt 3 1/2 ounces of the chocolate and keep warm enough to maintain a pourable consistency.

5. Whip the cream until stiff.

6. Combine your cream cheese, icing sugar, and vanilla in a separate bowl.

7. Stir the melted chocolate into the cream cheese mixture.

8. Fold your whipped cream into the cream cheese mixture.

9. Spoon your cheesecake mixture on top of the base, pressing down firmly onto the fruit. Smooth the top with a spatula.

10. Refrigerate before serving, for at least 2-3 hours (preferably overnight).

11. Arrange the remaining fruit on top of the cheesecake.

12. Melt your remaining chocolate and drizzle over the berries.

13. Serve and Enjoy!

Italian Tiramisu (Serves 2)

<u>Ingredients:</u>

<u>Cream:</u>

9 ounces of Mascarpone Cheese

1 3/4 ounces of Icing Sugar

2 tablespoons of Double Cream

2 tablespoons of Brandy

<u>Sponge:</u>

8 Trifle Sponge Fingers

2 tablespoons of Brandy

1 cup of Strong Cold Coffee

<u>Topping:</u>

3/4 ounce of Dark Chocolate Shavings

1 teaspoon of Cocoa Powder

Directions:

1. Cream your mascarpone together with the double cream, icing sugar, and brandy. Whisk until smooth.

2. Combine your cold coffee with 1 tablespoon of brandy.

3. Soak your trifle fingers in the coffee for a couple of seconds on each side. Start with half of your trifle fingers and arrange on the bottom of 2 small dessert bowls. You may need to cut some of the fingers in half to fit in better; fortunately, they'll bend once they're saturated with coffee.

4. Sprinkle chocolate shavings over the trifle sponge.

5. Spoon a quarter of the cream mixture into each bowl and spread out to fill the gaps between the sponge fingers.

6. Soak the remaining trifle fingers in the remaining coffee mixture and arrange on top of the cream.

7. Sprinkle with chocolate shavings, holding back a few shards to decorate the top.

8. Divide the remaining cream between the two bowls and spread out to a smooth surface.

9. Dust the top with cocoa powder and decorate with a few chocolate shavings.

10. Chill for at least a couple of hours before serving.

11. Serve and Enjoy!

Cranberry, Walnut & Chocolate Blondies (Serves 12)

<u>Ingredients:</u>

1 1/2 cups of Soft Brown Sugar

1 teaspoon of Vanilla Essence

1/2 cup of White Granulated Sugar

2 Eggs

2 cups of Plain Flour

1 1/2 teaspoons of Baking Powder

1 cup of Cranberries

1/2 cup of Walnuts

2 sticks of Butter

1 cup of Dark Chocolate chips

Directions:

1. Preheat your oven to 325 degrees.

2. Line a large-sized 9x13-inch deep baking pan with greaseproof paper.

3. Cream your butter together with the sugars (if your butter is straight from the fridge, you might want to soften it with 10-20 seconds in the microwave).

4. Beat in your eggs and vanilla essence.

5. Fold the flour and baking powder into your mixture.

6. Roughly chop the walnuts.

7. Stir the nuts, cranberries, and chocolate chips into the batter.

8. Spoon your batter into the baking pan and smooth the top with a spatula.

9. Bake for approximately 35 to 40 minutes, until a skewer, comes out clean and the top is starting to crack.

10. Cool in the tin for a few minutes before transferring to a wire rack.

11. Slice when cold.

12. Serve and Enjoy!

Fruit & Spice Bar (Serves 24)

<u>Ingredients:</u>

2 1/2 sticks of Butter

8 tablespoons of Golden Syrup

1 cup of Soft Brown Sugar

1 cup of Toasted Coconut Flakes

2 teaspoons of Mixed Spice

7 cups of Rolled Oats

1/2 cup of Raisins

1/2 cup of Glace Cherries (Quartered)

1/2 cup of Dried Cranberries

1/2 cup of Almonds (Roughly Chopped)

Zest of 1 Lemon (Finely Chopped)

Directions:

1. Preheat your oven to 380 degrees.

2. Melt your butter, sugar, and golden syrup in a large-sized glass bowl.

3. While your butter is melting, measure and chop the other ingredients.

4. Add about half of the oats, the spices, and the lemon zest into the melted butter mixture. Stir until the oats are coated in butter.

5. Add the fruit (unsticking any that have stuck together in the packet), almonds, and coconut. Mix thoroughly.

6. Add the remaining oats and stir until all the oats are coated in the butter mixture (i.e. no remaining white patches). The other ingredients should be fairly evenly distributed by this stage.

7. Line a deep-sided tray with greaseproof paper and press the mixture into the tray, smoothing with a spatula to ensure approximately even depth.

8. Bake for approximately 20 minutes, or until the surface is golden brown.

9. Allow it to cool in your tray until they are set hard enough to cut, then slice up and move to a wire rack to cool.

10. Serve and Enjoy!

Cherry Chocolate Coconut Bars (Serves 24)

Ingredients:

2 1/2 sticks of Butter

7 cups of Oats

1/3 cup of Molasses Sugar

2/3 cup of Soft Brown Sugar

1/2 cup of Maple Syrup

1 cup of Dark Chocolate Chips

1 cup of Cherries

1 cup of Desiccated Coconut

Directions:

1. Preheat your oven to 400 degrees.

2. Melt the butter, sugar, and golden syrup in a large-sized bowl.

3. While the butter is melting, quarter your cherries.

4. Stir about half of the oats and the coconut into the melted butter mixture.

5. Add the cherries and chocolate and mix until the cherries are evenly distributed. The chocolate will melt.

6. Add the remaining oats and stir until all your oats are coated in butter/chocolate mixture.

7. Line a deep-sided tray with greaseproof paper and press the mixture into the tray, smoothing with a spatula to ensure approximately even depth.

8. Bake for approximately 25 minutes until the top begins to brown.

9. Allow it to cool in the tray until they are set hard enough to cut. Slice up and move to a wire rack to cool completely.

10. Serve and Enjoy!

Conclusion

Thanks for reading my book. I hope this guide on Intermittent Fasting has provided you with all the necessary information you needed to get going. Don't put off getting started. The sooner you begin, the sooner you'll start to notice an improvement in your health and well-being. While results may vary, they will come if you stick to the information found in this book.

If you still have any unanswered questions I suggest checking out one of the resource sites or apps I discussed earlier. When I first got started learning about intermittent fasting these sites had all the answers I needed. They were truly an invaluable resource to have at my disposal. I believe in always trying to expand one's base of knowledge. I implore you to check out some of the books I suggested as they are all filled with great information. Don't be afraid to switch up your fasting methods if the first one you try isn't an ideal fit. I bounced around when I first started out before eventually settling on a plan that I felt comfortable with.

Good luck. I wish you nothing but the best!

www.ingramcontent.com/pod-product-compliance
Lightning Source LLC
Chambersburg PA
CBHW050911260726

48660CB00001B/138